Sports Medicine: Practical Guidelines for General Practice

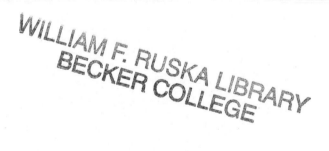

This book is dedicated to
Clodagh, Lucy, Yvonne and Chloe

Sports Medicine
Practical Guidelines for General Practice

Domhnall MacAuley MD MRCGP MICGP
MFPHMI FISM DPH DRCOG DipSpMed DSM

Hillhead Family Practice and The Queen's
University of Belfast

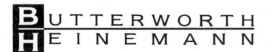
BUTTERWORTH
HEINEMANN

OXFORD AUCKLAND BOSTON JOHANNESBURG MELBOURNE NEW DELHI

Butterworth-Heinemann
Linacre House, Jordan Hill, Oxford OX2 8DP
225 Wildwood Avenue, Woburn, MA 01801-2041
A division of Reed Educational and Professional Publishing Ltd

ℛ A member of the Reed Elsevier plc group

First published 1999

© Reed Educational and Professional Publishing Ltd 1999

British Library Cataloguing in Publication Data
A catalogue record for this book is available from the British Library

ISBN 0 7506 3730 7

Typeset by Keyword Typesetting Services Ltd, Wallington, Surrey
Printed and bound in Great Britain by Biddles Ltd,
Guildford and King's Lynn

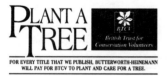

Contents

Preface   vii

1   Exercise: a historical perspective   1
2   Benefits of exercise   11
3   Promoting activity   28
4   Background physiology   42
5   Exercise for older people   53
6   Children and exercise   64
7   Treating minor injuries   70
8   Emergencies   85
9   Head injury   98
10 Spine and neck injury   103
11 Injuries of the upper limb   111
12 Injuries of the abdomen, groin, hip and thigh   124
13 Injuries of the lower leg   137
14 Injuries of the foot   166
15 Taping and injection   172
16 The team doctor   180
17 The doctor on tour   193
18 Acclimatisation   199
19 Outdoor and mountain pursuits   206
20 Exercise and illness   211
21 Dermatological problems   230
22 Women and sport   237
23 Diet and sport   247
24 Drugs in sport   257
Appendix: useful addresses   270

Index   274

Preface

General practice is where almost all sports medicine takes place. Almost every injury presents first in general practice and patients attend almost every day with sports-related problems. Patients also frequently ask about the benefits of exercise, how to get fit, or if physical activity can influence heart disease, diabetes, asthma or osteoporosis. This book was written to provide practical guidance on the managment of common injuries and advice on the relationship between health and exercise. It is designed for everyday use in the consulting room, to provide the answers to commonly-asked questions and offer a plan for the treatment of injuries in primary care.

The book addresses the most important topics we meet in practice and excludes rare or unusual conditions. It is not a specialist text, but is a guide to the management of common problems. It includes summary information for doctors and advice sheets for patients, and focuses on those areas that are of particular relevance to the team or touchline doctor.

No one could write such a book without considerable help from friends and colleagues. My fellow general practitioners and, more importantly my patients, helped mould this text by indicating what is important, and what is not, what they need to know and what is irrelevant, and what is of practical rather than purely academic interest. The information included is a distillation of advice, guidance and information obtained over many years. I have tried to credit all those I quote but there will be many others whose ideas I have heard, whose techniques I have integrated into my work and whose thoughts I have rehearsed so often that they have become my own. Forgive me if you recognise your ideas and I have forgotten where I first heard them.

Patients are only interested in keeping well or getting better. I hope that you can see their influence throughout the book. My colleagues have kept my feet on the ground and I wish to thank in particular my partners, Joe Dugan, Grainne Bonner and Siobhan McEntee. I have learned a lot from my friends in the British Association of Sport and Medicine, and especially colleagues Ian Corry, Michael Cullen, Martin Cunningham, Barbara Fair, Mark Hampton, Paul McCormack, Richard Nicholas, Bruce Thompson, Michael Webb and our mentor, Robin Harland. Others who have influenced my practice include, Ian Adams, Richard Budgett, Chuck Eaton, Maria Fiatarone, Peter Fricker, John Lloyd Parry, Donald McLeod, Nic Maffuli, Moira O'Brien, Peter Thomas, Dan Tunstall Pedoe, Malcolm Read, Peter Sperryn, Brian Walker, and Arnie Scheller and his team in Boston. Alun Evans has been an inspiration in my research.

1 Exercise: an historical perspective

The benefits of physical activity have been known since the earliest times. Of course, those advantages were more immediate when those who could run fastest, jump highest and throw furthest with most accuracy were those who survived. Darwin introduced the concept of the survival of the fittest in his *On the Origin of the Species* in 1859, in which he stated '... there must in every case be a struggle for existence, either one individual with another of the same species, or with individuals of distinct species, or with the physical conditions of life'. Life is rather different now and contemporary threats to the survival of humanity are much more subtle so that the risks of physical inactivity are less immediate. Modern life is almost devoid of any physical activity as we have eliminated the physical and active component from almost every occupation and household chore. This change in the pattern of our daily lives has been dramatic with the automation and mechanisation of almost all manufacturing processes and transport. Even a century ago, a third of the energy expended in US factories and farms was supplied by muscle power as compared with only 1% today. Evolution has not caught up, however, and we still possess the primitive biological response to fright, flight and fight together with all the associated biochemical and hormonal reactions. It is ironic that while we have taken the physical component out of almost every occupation we have invented a new phenomenon to take its place called 'exercise'. The physical activity that would have been an integral component of normal everyday life in the past, is now a planned, organised and structured activity during leisure time. We even medicalise physical activity to the extent that we have introduced exercise prescription schemes.

The history of physical activity

Tomb drawings in early Eastern civilisations provide us with the first evidence of the importance of physical development. Even in primitive society physical culture was important, not necessarily valued as a form of exercise, and certainly not for health benefits, it was often ritualised into dance. The earliest records of a link between exercise and medicine are from ancient China where, around 2500 BC, Hua T'o, a legend in Chinese surgery, encouraged exercises modelled on the movement of animals, principally the tiger. Kung Fu, which we now associate with violent combat, also had a medical origin as it began as a form of medical gymnastics. This medical gymnastics may in turn have been adapted from Yoga practised on the Indian subcontinent.

Most people associate the early Greek physicians with sport and exercise. The best known of these Greek physicians was Hippocrates (490–370BC) a doctor and teacher on the island of Cos and author of many treatises on health [1]. Modern medicine, and general practice in particular, echoes many of the principles of Hippocrates and the Greek School, placing the emphasis on the psychological background to illness, understanding patients within their own environment and the integration of the science and art of medicine. But the Greeks also emphasised the importance of physical well-being, fitness and a healthy active lifestyle. The well-known phrase 'mens sana in corpore sano', which defines the Greek ideal of physical and mental health, has almost become a mantra for protagonists of physical activity. Although often attributed to Plato, a contemporary of Hippocrates, it is actually taken from later work by Juvenal although it may describe a general philosophy of the time.

In ancient Greece, physical activity was an integral part of education and most education took place at the gymnasium. Plato's Academy was named after Akademos, a gymnasium, and Aristotle's school was located at Lyceum, another gymnasium. There was a long tradition of Greek athletics, pre-dating even Homer's Iliad, which described the funeral games for Patroclus (7th century BC), and Greek youth was encouraged to take part in organised games: gymnastics, boxing and wrestling in particular. Many early Greek sculptures, reliefs and archaeological exhibits depict sport, the best known being the discus thrower of Myron and the bronze statue of an athlete (circa 340 BC) in the National Archaeology Museum in Athens. The athlete personified the Greek ideal of bodily health, but although young Greeks were encouraged to be athletic, they were also encouraged in the arts and in the development of the mind. In Plato's Republic (c. 429-347 BC) the treatise on education suggests, 'And so we may venture to assert that anyone who can produce the best blend of the physical and intellectual sides of education and apply them to the training of character is producing harmony in a far more important sense than any pure musician'.

While physical health and gymnastic activity were important in education, they also had a wider role in health so that exercise was seen as a means of treating disease and disability and medical treatment included guidelines on diet and daily exercise. Exercise was also recognised for its public health benefits, but in Athens, Sparta and other city states, while sport may have been important for health, the advantages gained though physical fitness were essential for the citizen army [2]. Greece was in an almost constant state of war and physical fitness was greatly linked to military skills, important for both physical combat and rapid deployment of troops.

We are all familiar with the background to the Olympic Games, but there were originally four major athletic festivals, the Panhellenic Games at Olympia, Delphi, Isthmia and Nemea, and there were many local athletic festivals such as the Panathenaic Festival at Athens. These major festivals were held every four years but that at Olympia was the most important. The athletes competing at these games came at first from the upper social classes but in an uncanny parallel to the evolution of the modern Olympics, this changed. Prizes became valuable and athletes could afford to commit themselves full-time; thus the professional athlete was born. There was a conflict between those professional athletes and those who promoted sport and physical culture for health, and indeed the great philosophers held the professional athlete in low esteem. Hippocrates states in *Nutriment* [3]: 'The condition (diathesis) of the athlete is not natural. A healthy state (hexis) is superior to all'. He encouraged moderation and later Galen quoted Hippocrates in stating: 'Excessive and sudden filling or emptying or warming or chilling or otherwise stirring the body is dangerous ... any excess is hostile to nature' [4].

Galen, although Greek (c. 200–129 BC), spent many years studying medicine in Asia Minor, practised in Alexandria, and eventually settled in Rome where he was renowned as a physician. He acted as a 'team physician' to the gladiators and athletes and later served as a personal physician to Marcus Aurelius. He wrote many works on medicine, philosophy, rhetoric and grammar and an extensive essay on gymnastic exercises in a major work on health (*De Sanitate Tuenda*). He promoted moderate exercise for the health of both body and mind but had little regard for professional athletes and encouraged young men to study the arts rather than become athletes, stating '. . . while athletes are exercising their profession, their body remains in a dangerous condition, but when they give up their profession they fall into a condition more powerless still; as a fact, some die shortly afterward, others live for little time, but do not arrive at old age'. He also states, 'Athletes live a life quite contrary to the precepts of hygiene, and I regard their mode of living as a regime far more favourable to illness than to health'. Galen also quoted Hippocrates, who considered that professional athletes trained to excess, 'the perfect condition which these fellows strive for is dangerous', and advised, 'to keep well, avoid too much food, too little toil'.

There was a considerable disagreement between the athletic trainers, known as paedotribes, and medical opinion. The professional trainers learned practical physiology and the principles of athletic training empirically, and medical philosophers who considered that their knowledge was superior did not always approve. It is interesting to review the terminology used; 'health science' was attributed to the trainers, while 'hygiene' was taught by the physicians. Galen, however, believed that there was one single comprehensive science of care of the body, which was divided into therapy for the ill and maintenance of health in the healthy [5]. He encouraged moderation so there was balance between the body and mind, sport and the arts and stated, 'One of these arts, then, a young man should take up and practise, unless his mind is utterly brutish; and preferably the best art among them, which is, as we claim, medicine'.

Roman Empire and afterwards

The health benefits of exercise continued to be promoted during the Roman Empire and while physical fitness remained an essential military skill it was also a component of dietetics, a branch of medicine that included regulation of food and drink, exercise and bathing. Bathing was prescribed not only for maintenance of health but also as a means of curing illness [6]. Health advice was often provided by physical trainers at the baths, and medical treatment was available from doctors who practiced in the vicinity. The baths varied from small private buildings to large municipal sport and social centres where citizens could undertake exercise for sport and health. There was a difference, however, between the attitudes of the Greeks and the Romans who did not enjoy participating in multisport festivals. During the Dark Ages the Church became a dominant influence and 'body culture' fell into disrepute so that scholarly, monastic aestheticism became more important [7]. Physical education was kept solely for the preparation of knights and warriors. In Britain, sport was not an easy companion to Puritanism: the reading from the pulpit of *The Book of Sports*, which discussed sports and activities allowed on the Sabbath in 1618, during the reign of James I, highlighted the changing attitudes and sport only became acceptable after the decline of Puritanism. With these changing attitudes, sport was not only encouraged for the physical benefits but also for the benefit of the soul: a form of Christian–Judaic morality [8]. In contrast to the Dark Ages, exercise then became a practical manifestation of religious practice with the arrival of the 'muscular Christians' and as sport evolved it became, not so much a means to an end, but an end in itself [9].

Sport, as we now know it, evolved in the mid-Victorian era. Up to then, sports and games were mostly played in local communities, had little need of written rules, and sporting activity was often associated with religious festivals and seasonal celebrations. Boxing or prize fighting was popular with celebrated heroes such as the legendary Jack Broughton, and competition between professional watermen was common, leading to the oldest surviving fixture in the sporting calendar: the Doggett's Coat and Badge, a rowing race. Major rowing competitions had huge support and when Harry Clasper, a famous Geordie rower, died in 1870, a crowd of between 100,000 and 130,000 lined the streets at his funeral. Normal competitive behaviour had evolved to become a huge popular spectacle [10].

Exercise, health and the first studies of the medical benefits

Rowing was one of the earliest sports to have formal rules and became the model for many investigations of intense physical activity. Galen's view that vigorous physical activity was harmful persisted, even into the 19th century, and it was this perception that prompted Morgan [11] to study the health of those who had participated in the University Boat Race. He studied longevity and subsequent health of university oarsmen who had participated in the first forty years (1829–1869) of the Oxford and Cambridge boat race and found that the average length of life for each oarsman, assuming an age of 20 at the time of the boat race, was of a further 42.2 years. The normal expectation of life at that time, based on contemporary English Life tables constructed by William Farr, compiler of abstracts for the Registrar General, was of a further 40 years. The extent to which life exceeded expectation was 2.2 years. Of course this comparison was invalid as it was confounded by social class factors and Morgan should have taken controls from the contemporary student population but it is still an important study. Incidentally, he found that Oxford University crews lived longer than Cambridge crews (Oxford 3.7 years and Cambridge 0.7 years of life longer than expected). The contemporary view on intense physical activity is illustrated in Morgan's text, *University Oars*, in which the Reverend Charles Wordsworth, afterwards Bishop of St Andrew's, is quoted: '... in those days we used to be told that no man in a "racing" [sic] boat could expect to live to the age of thirty'. Rowing retained the interest of the medical profession and a further study [12] of the longevity of oarsmen who rowed in the boat race from 1829 to 1928 concluded, '... that over the whole period of investigation the mortality experience of university oarsmen was appreciably superior to that of assured lives of their own generation, but that of late years this relative superiority had been shown to diminish'. Medical opinion had changed and physiologists and physicians felt the danger had been greatly exaggerated. Hartley, the author of this study, believed that most would take the view that, '... no young man will injure himself by rowing provided that his organs are sound and that he has previously undergone a proper course of training'.

Dr Louis Dublin [13] studied the life histories of 38,269 graduates from 10 of the eastern colleges in the United States and found the mortality of college graduates was 91% of that of USA men. In reviewing the medical histories of athletes and honours graduates in particular, he found that honours graduates had lower mortality. Rook [14] confirmed this finding in a study of Cambridge sportsmen in which intellectuals lived longer by a period averaging about 1.5 years, although he conceded that this difference may have been due to chance. The hazards of rowing have continued to exercise medical minds and in an analysis of the life expectancy of college oarsmen at Harvard and Yale from 1882 to

1902, rowers lived longer than controls by 6.35 years at Yale and 6.24 years at Harvard [15]. Mortality due to heart disease has been studied in other sports. In a study of 355 men who had distinguished themselves in college football from 1901 to 1930, the cause of death was established in 87 cases, and in 25 of these it was due to coronary heart disease [16]. Those who had coronary heart disease participated in less vigorous exercise than the others and no-one who was vigorously active developed coronary heart disease.

James Mackenzie (1853–1925), the pioneer of general practice [17] who first described the polygraph, defended intense physical activity in sport and at work, at a time when severe exertion was considered harmful. He did not believe that exercise was harmful and challenged a contemporary Cambridge physician to send him a case where exercise had caused damage to the heart. He is also indirectly associated with the Framingham study, which was to become one of the most important cohort studies of cardiovascular disease and which strongly supports the epidemiological link between physical inactivity and cardiovascular disease. Paul Dudley White visited James Mackenzie in St Andrews in 1918 and later began the Framingham study in 1922. It was much later before Abrahams, in his major review in 1951, stated that strenuous exercise had no immediate ill effect on the normal heart [18]. But perhaps it was in the north of Ireland that the cardiovascular benefits of exercise were first noted when Samuel Black of Newry, County Down, who described his first case of angina in 1794, noted the beneficial influence of physical activity and suggested that walking was preferable to every other mode of exercise [19].

Exercise and occupations

The relationship between physical activity at work and coronary heart disease was to come to prominence later. One of the earliest comparisons between sedentary work and active work is that of the Sanitary Circumstances of Tailors in London [20] which described the work patterns of tailors, and concluded that mortality among tailors was much higher than that of agricultural labourers, and that they were '... a feeble and sensitive class, and in only a very small minority of cases give evidence of health equal to those engaged in many other indoor occupations'. While physical activity at work was the pattern of the lower classes, coronary heart disease was at that time an affliction of the upper social classes, as observed by Osler [21] in 1910. He commented on the '. . . remarkable fact with which we are all familiar, that angina pectoris is an affection of the better classes, and not often seen except in private practice'. This pattern was further illustrated in the Occupational Mortality Supplement for 1930–32 which recorded a considerable excess of coronary mortality in the men of social classes I and II. Morris [22] quotes the Registrar General (*Decennial Supplement*, 1938) who suggested that sedentariness of work and nervous and dietary factors may have been involved. Thus may the theory that physical activity at work was related to coronary heart disease have had its origins in British social class data indicating that coronary disease mortality in the professional and business class was double that in unskilled workers.

One of the earliest epidemiological studies of cardiovascular disease incidence [23] noted that mortality from acute coronary occlusion was highest among men in the business and professional groups particularly among professional men aged 55–64 years in whom the estimated mortality was considerably higher than among other groups, especially manual workers. Epidemiological evidence suggesting a link with physical activity at work began to emerge and although it is possible that these results may have been due to variations in the characteristics of the subjects, i.e. self selection, these early studies, even with potential methodological errors, drew the attention of epidemiologists to the beneficial effects of physical activity and were the forerunners of many subsequent investigations.

Limits to performance

Athletic performance has improved over the ages and no world record established before 1980 still exists. More recently, however, the rate of improvement in performance has slowed so that it took until 1991 before Bob Beamon's 23-year-old long jump record of 8.9 metres was surpassed and the 200 m record stood for 17 years before Michael Johnson broke it in 1996. Performance in power events has not only failed to improve but there has been a noticeable overall decline, although this may in part be due to increased efforts to detect drug abuse. It may be that we are now approaching a limit to human performance. Some further improvements may be achieved through the introduction of new technologies.

Technological advances have had a dramatic influence on events such as the pole vault, which now requires a completely different technique, and in the javelin where the regulations have been changed. Cycling time-trial records have been rewritten as much through design innovation as through improvements in physiological performance. The surface consistency of athletic tracks can be manipulated to improve the speed of sprinters and the preparation of Astroturf pitches can change the speed of field hockey.

Understanding the physiological and psychological background to performance has also helped change the training and preparation of athletes. Participants in many sports now include plyometric training to take advantage of the elastic component of muscle contraction and use psychological preparation to achieve performance advantage.

It is very difficult to quantify those improvements that can be attributed to drugs or medical manipulation. Altitude training gave those athletes who could afford it a legal advantage, and laboratory evidence confirms the benefits gained in performance through blood doping and erythropoietin. More recently published scientific evidence has demonstrated the benefits gained through the use of anabolic steroids, advantages that have been recognised by athletes for many years.

It is difficult to predict the changes that may occur in future athletic performance. Overall, people are becoming taller, heavier and stronger. Nations that used not take part in international competition are now taking the majority of medals in certain events. Who knows what technological advances or medical manipulation will change the face of sport in the future?

References

1 Lyons AS, Petrucelli RJ. *Medicine. An Illustrated History*. Abradale Press, Harry N Abrams Inc., New York, 1978.
2 McIntosh PCI. Sport in society. In *Sports Medicine* (Williams JGP, Sperryn PN Eds) Edward Arnold, London, 1976.
3 Hippocrates. Nutriment Section xxxiv, *loeb class*. lib. 1,355.
4 Robinson RS. *Sources for the History of Greek Athletics*. R S Robinson, Cincinnati, 1955.
5 Smith WD. *The Hippocratic Tradition*. Cornell University Press, 1979.
6 Jackson R. *Doctors and Diseases in the Roman Empire*. British Museum Publications, London, 1988.
7 Williams, JGP. *Medical Aspects of Sport and Physical Fitness*. Pergamon Press, London, 1965.
8 Loy JW, Kenyon GS. *Sport, Culture, and Society*. Macmillan, New York, 1969.

9 Holt R. *Sport and the British. A modern history*. Clarendon Press, Oxford, 1989.
10 Dodd C. *The Story of World Rowing*. Stanley Paul, London, 1992.
11 Morgan JE. *University Oars*. Macmillan, London, 1873.
12 Hartley PHS, Llewellyn GF. The longevity of oarsmen; a study of those who rowed in the Oxford and Cambridge Boat Race from 1829–1928. *BMJ* 1939; **1**: 657–662.
13 Dublin LI. *Statistical Bulletin*. Metropolitan Life Insurance Co., August, 1932.
14 Rook A. An investigation into the longevity of Cambridge oarsmen. *BMJ* 1954; **1**: 773–777.
15 Prout C. Life expectancy of college oarsmen. *JAMA* 1972; **220**: 1709–11.
16 Pomeroy WC, White PD. Coronary heart disease in former football players. *JAMA* 1958: **167**: 711–14.
17 Mairs A. *Sir James Mackenzie MD 1853–1926*. Royal College of General Practitioners, London, 1989.
18 Abrahams A. Physical Exercise. Its clinical associations. *Lancet* 1951: **i**, 1133–1137, 1187–1192.
19 Black S. *Clinical and Pathological Reports*. Alexander and Wilkinson, Newry, 1819.
20 Smith E. Report on the Sanitary Conditions of Tailors in London. *Report of the Medical Officer, The Privy Council*, 1864: 416–30.
21 Osler W. Angina pectoris. *Lancet* 1910: **i**, 697–702.
22 Morris JN, Heady JA, Raffle PAB, Roberts CG, Parks JW. Coronary heart disease and physical activity at work. *Lancet* 1953; **ii**, 1053–1057, 1111–1120.
23 Hedley OF. Analysis of 5,116 deaths reported as due to acute coronary occlusion in Philadelphia 1933–37. *Public Health Rep* 1939; June: 1972–1012.

2 Benefits of exercise

Exercise has many well documented benefits to physical and mental well-being. The main focus of research has been on the cardiovascular system and in particular the prevention and treatment of coronary heart disease [1–3], stroke [4], and the modification of risk factors including the various lipid subfractions [5]. It is also of value in the prevention and treatment of hypertension [6] and asthma [7]. The Position Statement of the American College of Sports Medicine, summarises the evidence that exercise may aid a calorie controlled diet in weight reduction [8] and exercise may also improve tissue sensitivity to insulin, of particular value in adult onset diabetes [9]. Fit people, in general, suffer less back pain [10] and physical activity may also help to maintain or even increase bone density. Indeed, regular exercise could reduce the risk of post menopausal osteoporotic fracture by up to 50% resulting in 20,000 less hip fractures per year in the United Kingdom [11].

Regular physical activity has been associated with lower rates of some cancers, and may reduce all cancer mortality [12,13]. Exercise has been shown to reduce the risk of colon cancer [14,15] and although very little is known about the relationship between physical activity and protection from malignancy, there is evidence from one study that not only does physical activity offer some protection against colon cancer but that physical activity during college years also appeared to protect against some neoplasia of the reproductive organs [16].

The most impressive findings have been the reduction in deaths from cardiovascular disease (and indeed all-cause mortality) associated with both physical activity and physical fitness. This is of particular importance in the United Kingdom where coronary heart disease is the leading cause of death, responsible for about 170,000 deaths or one quarter of all deaths annually. It has been estimated that about one third of ischaemic heart disease incidents could be avoided by appropriate physical activity, a factor which could have major implications in general practice. We are unsure, however, of the exact mechanism of these benefits and it may be that the cardiovascular benefits are due to the effect on risk factors. The major known risk factors are hypertension, cigarette smoking and raised cholesterol, and exercise may directly or indirectly affect these or related factors. There is considerable evidence for a beneficial effect on lipid profile, not only through a reduction in serum cholesterol triglycerides but also by elevating HDL cholesterol, which appears to have a protective effect [17,18]. Exercise has also been shown to have a beneficial effect on hypertension and a sustained exercise programme can help reduce blood pressure [19]. More recently, the focus has expanded to include the metabolic syndrome, known as Syndrome X, which includes hypertension, insulin resistance, glucose intolerance and hyperlipidaemia. Exercise can improve insulin sensitivity and this may be a key step in reducing obesity, hypertension and modifying lipid profile. Exercise can, of course, aid weight reduction [20]. There are also documented changes in blood clotting factors [21]. Well documented physiological changes include a reduction in heart rate and an increase in end diastolic volume.

The overwhelming evidence pointing to a relationship between physical inactivity and cardiovascular disease has lead to a re-evaluation of the importance of the traditional risk factors and physical inactivity is considered to be a factor of equal importance to the established risk factors of hypertension, smoking and elevated cholesterol [22]. More importantly, physical inactivity is an independent risk factor in studies across many different populations and the effect persists even after adjustment for possible confounding variables.

Exercise is now also considered to be an important component of secondary prevention and graded exercise is an integral part of many cardiac rehabilitation programmes. There is evidence from a number of different studies, and a meta-analysis of post-myocardial infarction exercise training has shown a significant reduction in deaths [23].

Physical activity, physical fitness and cardiovascular disease

An active lifestyle protects against coronary heart disease and the beneficial effects are dose related to the intensity of physical activity. With the accumulation of findings from many studies there is good evidence that the relationship is causal. Most of us have some recollection of the early landmark studies on both sides of the Atlantic. In the United Kingdom, Morris and his colleagues performed epidemiological studies of post office workers, bus drivers and bus conductors. Admittedly there were possible confounding variables in these early studies but they did draw attention to the beneficial effect of physical activity. In the United States, Paffenbarger and his co-workers also found that physical activity during work or leisure reduced the risk of heart attack. This finding was subsequently confirmed in many studies including the Framingham study.

Morris and Paffenbarger were the two key early investigators who focused attention on physical activity, particularly at work. In one of the first studies Morris and colleagues [24] compared two groups of workers with contrasting work patterns, bus drivers with conductors and postmen with office post workers, and demonstrated a difference in mortality patterns. The drivers of double-decker buses were more likely to die suddenly from coronary thrombosis than conductors, and the office workers died more often from cardiac infarction than the more active postmen. Of course, these studies were subject to many potential sources of bias, particularly in self selection to the various occupations, a factor which was confirmed in later studies which showed that the drivers were taller and heavier with higher cholesterol values [25]. Although open to criticism, these were landmark studies in the evolution of the epidemiological evidence of the beneficial relationship between physical activity and heart disease. Subsequent studies showed that ischaemic myocardial fibrosis was more common in men with light occupations than those with active and heavy occupations [26]. Morris and his group also explored the physical activity pattern of civil servants in what has become known as the Whitehall study. They asked 16,882 male executive grade civil servants aged 40–64 across Britain to record all their activities over a weekend and followed this cohort for a number of years. The findings were remarkable and those who had been vigorously physically active were only about one third as likely to develop coronary disease as those who did not [27]. Following this cohort for a longer period, they showed that those who had taken part in vigorous sports during the initial survey in 1968–70 had less than half the incidence of coronary heart disease than their inactive colleagues [28]. The protective effect was only present in those who were vigorously active, defined as energy expenditure of 7.5 kcal per min [29].

At the same time, Ralph Paffenbarger was researching the benefits of work related physical activity. He studied a particularly active group of dock workers, the cargo handlers. At that time all loading and unloading of ships was undertaken manually and this group had an exceptionally high energy expenditure. Their very active lifestyle had a protective effect against cardiovascular disease [30] with a lower incidence of sudden death and overall lower death rate. He also studied the protective effect of physical activity in a very different population group: graduates of Harvard. In this, known as the Harvard alumni study [31], the risk of first heart attack was inversely related to energy expenditure in physical activity so that the risk of first heart attack was 64% higher in men who expended less than 2,000 kcal per week in leisure time physical activity. An interesting finding of this study was the importance of current levels of activity and that it was current physical activity that exerted the protective effect. Among those who had been active in the past, exercise had to be continued to maintain the protective effect but those who had been inactive in the past, and took up exercise, gained the advantages associated with physical activity. The benefits of exercise were independent of factors including smoking, obesity, weight gain, hypertension and family history. Later, they demonstrated that deaths from all causes were significantly lower, and not just deaths from coronary artery disease [32]. In contrast to the study on dock workers, the energy expenditure was much lower, but still those who were more active were at an advantage. Death rates were one quarter to one third lower among those expending 2,000 kcal per week or more in leisure time physical activity, a level which corresponds to 5 hours brisk walking (at 7 km per hour) or 3.5 hours running (at 9 km per hour) per week. The benefits of activity were seen among those who were active, independent of blood pressure, cigarette smoking, obesity or family history.

The Framingham heart study [33], perhaps the most comprehensive epidemiological study of cardiovascular risk factors, also demonstrated the benefits of physical activity in terms of cardiovascular mortality and morbidity. More importantly, however, it showed a relationship with moderate activity.

While the evidence from these cohort studies is convincing, they have one particular limitation in common, in that they relate the long-term outcome to a single baseline measure of physical

activity. Habits may change, and health and domestic circumstances alter, so that the single baseline measurement may not
be an accurate reflection of long-term patterns. There may also
be an interrelationship between activity and other risk factors. A
more recent study [34], attempted to take these issues into consideration and not only confirmed these findings but showed that
in taking these issues into account, the protective effect of physical activity appeared to be stronger.

From the early studies of Morris and Paffenbarger, the volume
of research expanded greatly and this evidence was collated in
two major reviews. In the first of these [35], which gathered high
quality evidence from 43 studies of physical activity, there was a
consistent inverse association between physical activity and coronary heart disease. These 43 studies were selected from a list of
121 articles representing at least 54 studies and the selection criteria were rigorous so that only those studies that qualified were
included. In order to be included it was essential that incident
cases could be separated from prevalence cases, and that incidence rates, relative rates, odds ratios, mortality ratios or a
regression analysis were available. This left 36 cohort studies,
three mortality studies, and four case-controlled studies, although
the information available was generally limited to employed
North American and European men. Using accepted criteria for
causation [36], they concluded that these studies confirmed that
lower cardiovascular mortality was associated with physical
activity. Using the more sophisticated methodology of meta-analysis, a later study [37] confirmed the increased risk associated
with inactivity and postulated that the risk of heart attack was
increased by a factor of 1.9 in those who were inactive. Many of
the included studies used different outcome measures such as
coronary heart disease incidence or death, myocardial infarction
with or without sudden death, angina and congestive heart failure, but the relationship was consistent and indeed the higher
quality studies tended to show a higher relative risk. Overall
they concluded that physical inactivity was a potentially modifiable risk factor and one that should have greater emphasis.

The energy threshold

While physical activity indeed has a beneficial effect, many
researchers were interested to know how much physical activity
was necessary to achieve this advantage. Many of our patients are

also keen to know how much exercise is necessary. The early studies of Paffenbarger and Morris showed great variation in exercise related energy expenditure but as the research evidence evolved many studies showed similar results but at different levels of activity. It appears from the available evidence, from large well controlled prospective studies in particular, that the beneficial effects are dose related and that starting to exercise, even in later life, is beneficial.

Measuring physical activity is difficult and researchers have used many different methods in questionnaires, diaries, cumulative work activity and physical fitness measures. The early studies used mainly measures of physical activity at work only, but the physical activity component of most occupations has now gone, and most exercise is undertaken during leisure time. From the early studies, it appeared that there was a threshold effect. Morris and his colleagues [27] found that 30 minutes of vigorous physical activity per day at an energy expenditure 7.5 kcal per min was required to demonstrate a reduction in cardiovascular mortality. Such activity is equivalent to an energy expenditure of 225 kcal per day and an accumulative total of 1,575 kcal per week. Similarly, Paffenbarger found that there was a reduction in mortality from a weekly accumulative energy expenditure of less than 500 kcal to more than 2,000 kcal. With an expenditure of more than 2,000 kcal there was little additional benefit [32]. Other studies pointed to a similar energy expenditure. Moderate exercise is also effective [38], so that activities such as walking, cycling and gardening are associated with a reduced risk and vigorous exercise gave no additional benefit. In some studies as little as 20 minutes of walking per day would be necessary [39] or an accumulated energy expenditure of at least 1,000 kcal per week in moderate intensity activity [40].

Moderate physical activity clearly offers some protective effect [41] but there is also a dose–response relationship with increasing expenditure [42] with a gradient of risk across activity or fitness levels [43].

Physical fitness

Many reviewers confuse physical activity and physical fitness, but they are not equivalent and may have a different pathway in their relationship with cardiovascular disease. The definition of physical activity is of 'bodily movement produced by skeletal muscles that results in energy expenditure', while 'physical fitness is a set of attributes that people have or achieve that are related to their ability to perform physical activity'. Physical activity represents the accumulated activity in both work and leisure time and is usually assessed using a questionnaire [44]. Few studies include a measure of physical fitness and there are even fewer high quality studies comparing physical fitness, measured either in performance on an ergometer or by measurement of VO_2 max, to later risk of heart attack. In those that have measured physical fitness, there has been an associated subsequent reduction in cardiovascular mortality.

While it is difficult to separate the effects of physical activity and physical fitness, the relationship between these two factors and cardiovascular disease has been investigated [45]. In this study it was physical fitness level, and not the measure of physical activity, that appeared to be the independent protective factor. The inverse relationship between physical fitness and cardiovascular mortality remains after adjustment for possible confounding factors [41,46]. While activity and fitness may often be associated, physical activity is not always correlated with cardiovascular fitness [44,47,48], a factor with a major genetic influence.

A weakness of much of the research is that it focuses almost exclusively on men, middle-aged men in particular. In a recent large study, including both men and women, there were similar results confirming the inverse relationship between exercise and mortality [49] but this study also included details of other risk factors to compare their relative risk. The relative risks for hypertension and cholesterol were 1.3, but more interestingly, the relative risk of all-cause mortality due to low fitness (1.52) and cigarette smoking (1.65) were similar which suggests that becoming fit and ceasing smoking would be equally effective in reducing mortality. From this study we can also compare the protective effect of cardiorespiratory fitness and other risk factors in combination. Those in the high fitness group with multiple risk factors had lower death rates than those in the low fitness groups who had no other risk factors.

More recently, a study of 40,417 postmenopausal women confirmed that the benefits also applied to women, when they demonstrated that those who were most active had a longer lifespan. The relationship was related to the amount and intensity of activity but even those who exercised moderately only once per week had a 22% lower risk of death [50].

Exercise, lipids and lipoproteins

Cholesterol and lipid subfractions are known risk factors for cardiovascular disease, but those who are most active have lower levels and it may be that this link contributes to the lower cardiovascular mortality associated with physical activity [18]. This link may, however, be reduced when the statistical relationship is adjusted for covariates [51]. The combined evidence in a meta-analysis of 66 training studies showed, however, that those who were physically active had lower total cholesterol, triglycerides and LDL cholesterol with a higher level of HDL cholesterol. Comparing groups which are most active with sedentary controls may not tell the whole story, and when we examine population studies we find that the strength of the relationship is less than that seen in cross-sectional, case-control led and (to a lesser extent) in intervention studies [52]. In particular, differences in lipid levels between trained athletes and controls are much greater than those seen across populations.

The lipid component may be only one dimension of the risk relationship and it may be that the apolipoproteins (the peptide components of the lipoproteins which act as membrane receptor sites and cofactors for enzymes in lipoprotein metabolism) have a major role. Indeed, those patients with diagnosed coronary artery disease have significantly lower apoAI and apoAII. ApoAI is apolipoprotein associated with HDL cholesterol and may be more important in the development of coronary artery disease, while apoB is the apolipoprotein associated with LDL cholesterol. There is a relationship between physical activity and lipoprotein subfractions in cross-sectional studies comparing active and less active people and in training studies [53]. Lipoprotein (a) (the low density lipoprotein which has attracted recent interest because of its association with coronary heart disease) does not appear to be associated with physical activity.

The beneficial changes in lipids and lipoproteins associated with physical activity do not, however, appear to be seen in relation to physical fitness which suggests that the beneficial effect of physical fitness may be mediated through an alternative pathway.

Hypertension

There is a reduced risk of hypertension in those who are most active [54,55], with an inverse relationship between vigorous sports participation and hypertension [56], a relationship that is independent of age, body mass index (BMI) and fasting plasma insulin levels [57]. This inverse relationship may not be present at the highest levels of activity as demonstrated in the MRFIT [58] and British Regional Heart Study [59] which suggested a J-shaped curve. The findings from a meta-analysis of 25 longitudinal studies [60] is strong evidence, however, of lowered elevated systolic and diastolic blood pressure with exercise, and the relative risk in those who are least fit is 1.52 for hypertension when compared to those who are fittest [61]. There is also evidence from a controlled trial in those with high-normal blood pressure at baseline, that an intervention which included exercise reduced the risk of developing hypertension [62]. Exercise can lower systolic blood pressure by 11 mmHg and diastolic blood pressure by 8 mmHg in those with mild to moderate hypertension [60].

It is possible that the changes in blood pressure associated with exercise may be related to other factors including gender, BMI, intensity of exercise, duration of training and initial blood pressure, but notwithstanding these possible criticisms the consensus that exercise is of benefit has lead to guidelines for exercise prescription in hypertension Those who appear to benefit most are women, those with higher initial diastolic blood pressure, those who exercise at low intensity and those who make a long-term commitment to exercise. A recent review summarises the influence of physical exercise on blood pressure [63].

Fibrinogen

Physical activity also affects the blood clotting mechanism, plasma fibrinogen in particular. Fibrinogen is, of course, a known risk factor for cardiovascular disease [64,65], and the lower level associated with exercise is another possible mechanism for the reduction in cardiovascular mortality associated with physical activity. In epidemiological studies such as the Whitehall study [29], the Gothenburg study [66], the Caerphilly prospective heart disease study [67], the Scottish heart health study [68], and the ARIC study, lower fibrinogen levels were shown in those who were most active. In the MRC study [69], the vigorously active group had lower fibrinogen levels, even after adjustment for possible confounders such as age, smoking, alcohol, BMI and occupation, and in the Caerphilly prospective heart disease study [70], plasma fibrinogen was 0.24 g per litre lower in the more active group. The MRC group suggested that the lower levels of plasma fibrinogen may explain the reduction in cardiovascular mortality with physical activity, using in illustration the Necropsy study [26] where there was no difference in the degree of coronary artery atheroma in the different activity groups but there was a difference in the degree of coronary artery occlusion and large healed infarcts. A major review of the evidence [71] concluded that the reduction of plasma fibrinogen by about 0.4 g per litre with physical activity could mean a considerable reduction in the risk of coronary heart disease. This magnitude of plasma fibrinogen reduction should be seen in the context of an estimated 15% risk reduction with a decrease of just 0.1 g per litre in other work [72].

How much exercise?

The question that our patients really want answered is how much exercise is required to gain the protective effect. The evidence from most of the studies of physical activity is that there is a dose–response relationship and that the benefits are greatest in those who are vigorously active. There is of course evidence of a reduction in risk in those who are moderately active and this has coloured much of the recent advice on physical activity at community level. Public health bodies, particularly those in the United States, have used this evidence to change the generic health message and the global exercise prescription has changed. These guidelines are, to an extent, a pragmatic effort to find a compromise between a level of activity that has proven benefits, and one that can be undertaken by the majority of the population with minimum risk. The current advice is that we should all be physically active, above our baseline activities of daily living, to an equivalent calorie intake of 1000 kcal (4200 kJ) per week. This prescription is equivalent to 30–40 minutes of moderate physical activity on 5–7 days per week and, more importantly, the guidelines do not indicate that this activity should be of a sporting nature. The energy expenditure in many activities is equivalent so that achieving the moderate intensity and duration targets can include a wide variety of sport and leisure activities. The accumulated energy expenditure may be achieved from a variety of different activities which include the established aerobic types such as running, swimming, cycling and rowing, but may also be gained through tennis, football, golf and home-based activity such as gardening, DIY or washing the car. Even more revolutionary, and perhaps more acceptable to the general population, is the evidence that the exercise need not be continuous and that the energy targets, and the associated health benefits, can be gained from an aggregate of shorter bursts of activity rather than a single longer period [73].

A consensus development panel on physical activity and cardiovascular health [74] stated the following: 'All Americans should engage in regular physical activity at a level appropriate to their capacity, needs and interest. Children and adults alike should set a goal of accumulating at least 30 minutes of moderate intensity physical activity on most and preferably all days of the week. Most Americans have little or no physical activity in their daily lives and accumulating evidence indicates that physical inactivity is a major risk factor for cardiovascular disease. Even those who currently meet these daily standards may derive additional health and fitness benefit by becoming more physically active and accumulating more vigorous physical activity. For those with cardiovascular disease, cardiac rehabilitation programmes that combine physical activity with reduction in other risk factors should be more widely used.'

These are population guidelines and are a general prescription rather than an individually tailored message. The advice will vary for those who are young, active and healthy, and those who are older and less active. The more active group will benefit from greater energy expenditure in intensity and duration while more modest targets may be appropriate for others such as the older, disabled and less fit.

Current activity levels

Establishing figures for the proportion of the population which is active is difficult but many countries have attempted to do so. Comparing exact percentages between countries, and even within countries, is fraught with difficulty because surveys using different questionnaires, and even cultural interpretation of the same questionnaire can give vastly different results [75]. Data from studies in the United States and Canada suggest that 20% of the population exercise to vigorous intensity at a frequency likely to improve cardiovascular fitness, an additional 40% are active at a more moderate level, and 40% are completely sedentary. There is little difference in the proportion of men and women who are active to a moderate level, but men are more likely to be vigorously active. Similar figures are available from Australia, where those who are inactive tend to be older, less well educated, and to have lower incomes.

The most comprehensive and accurate data for physical activity participation in the United Kingdom is from the Allied Dunbar national fitness survey [76] and the Northern Ireland health and activity survey [77]. These surveys used an identical questionnaire which enabled researchers to collate comprehensive data on physical activity at work and at home and included information on intensity, frequency and duration which together give an accurate picture of population activity levels. Other studies which included a physical activity measurement were Heartbeat Wales [78,79], the Scottish heart health study [80], and the General Household Survey [81].

National data for England indicate that 14% of men and 4% of women are vigorously active for at 20 min on three occasions each week. In Northern Ireland, where data were collected using the same method, the corresponding figures are 21% and 6%. For exercise at moderate intensity, 49% of men and 41% of women are active on average on three occasions each week and in Northern Ireland 52% of men and 46% of women achieve this level of activity. Data from Scotland (which used a different method of measuring activity and may not be directly comparable) found that 14% of men and 10% of women were regularly active during leisure time. Other studies reflect intermediate levels of participation with over 40% of men and a variable proportion of women recorded as moderately active depending on the particular study.

Benefits of exercise: summary

- Lower mortality, even among those who are only moderately active
- Reduced risk of coronary artery disease
- Modifies lipid profile
- Lowers blood pressure
- Reduces risk of colon cancer

▶

- Helps prevent obesity
- Reduces risk of non-insulin-dependent diabetes mellitus
- Protects against osteoporosis
- Improves strength and helps reduce falls in the elderly
- Helps back pain
- May help asthma
- Improves mood and aids depression

References

1 Fentem P, Bassey J, Turnbull N. *The New Case for Exercise*. Health Education Authority, Sports Council, 1988.
2 Fentem PH, Bassey EJ. *The Case for Exercise*. Research Working Paper No 8, Sports Council, 1976.
3 Dargie HJ, Grant S. Exercise. *BMJ* 1991; **303**: 910–12.
4 Salonen JT, Puska P, Tuomilento J. Physical activity and risk of myocardial infarction, cerebral stroke and death. *Am J Epidemiol* 1982; **115**: 526–37.
5 Haskell WL. The influence of exercise training on plasma lipids and lipoproteins in health and disease. *Acta Med Scand* 1986; **711**: 25–37.
6 Fagard R. Habitual physical activity, training and blood pressure in normo- and hypertension. *Int J Sports Med* 1985; **6**: 57–67.
7 Bundgaard A. Asthma. *Sports Med* 1985; **2**: 254–66.
8 American College of Sports Medicine. Position Statement: Proper and improper weight loss programs. *Med Sci Sports Exer* 1983; **15** (ix).
9 Siscovick DS, Laporte RE, Newman JM. The disease-specific benefits and risks of physical activity and exercise. *Public Health Rep* 1985; **100**; 180–88.
10 Frymoyer JW. Back pain and sciatica. *N Engl J Med* 1988; **318**: 291–300.
11 Law MR, Wald NJ, Meade TW. Strategies for prevention of osteoporosis and hip fracture. *BMJ* 1991; **303**: 453–9.
12 Shephard RJ. Does exercise reduce all cancer death-rates? *Br J Sports Med* 1992; **26**: 125–28.
13 Shephard RJ. Physical activity and cancer. *Int J Sports Med* 1990; **11**: 413–20.
14 Vena JE, Graham S, Zielezny M, Swanson MK *et al.* Lifetime occupational exercise and colon cancer. *Am J Epidemiol* 1985; **122**: 357–365.
15 Powell KE, Casperson CJ, Koplan JP, Ford ES. Physical activity and chronic diseases. *Am J Clin Nutr* 1989; **49**: 999–1006.
16 Kohl HW, LaPorte RE, Blair SN. Physical activity and cancer. An epidemiological perspective. *Sports Med* 1988; **6**: 222–37.
17 Stefanick ML, Wood PD. Physical activity, lipid and lipoprotein metabolism and lipid transport. In *Physical Activity, Fitness and Health* (Bouchard C, Shepherd RJ, Stephens T) International Proceedings and Consensus statement. Champaign IL: Human Kinetics Publishers, 1994: 417–431.
18 MacAuley D. Exercise, cardiovascular disease and lipids. *Br J Clin Prac* 1993; **47**: 323–327.

19 American College of Sports Medicine. Physical activity, physical fitness and hypertension: position stand. *Med Sci Sports Exer* 1993; **25**: 1–10.

20 Blair SN. Evidence for the success of exercise in weight loss and control. *Ann Intern Med* 1993; **119**: 702–706.

21 MacAuley D, McCrum EE, Stott G *et al.* Physical activity, physical fitness, blood pressure, and fibrinogen in Northern Ireland Health. *J Epidemiol Commun Health* 1996; **50**: 258–263.

22 American Heart Association Committee on Exercise. *Circulation* 1992; **86**: 340–4.

23 Oldridge NB, Guyatt GH, Fischer ME, Rimm AA. Cardiac rehabilitation after myocardial infarction. *JAMA* 1988; **260**: 945–950.

24 Morris JN, Heady JA, Raffle PAB, Roberts CG, Parks JW. Coronary heart disease and physical activity at work. *Lancet* 1953; **ii**: 1053–57, 1111–20.

25 Oliver RM. Physique and serum lipids of young London busmen in relation to ischaemic heart disease. *Br J Ind Med* 1967; **24**: 181–8.

26 Morris JN, Crawford MD. Coronary heart disease and physical activity of work: evidence of a national necropsy survey. *BMJ* 1958; **511**: 1484–96.

27 Morris JN, Chave SPW, Adam C *et al.* Vigorous exercise in leisure time and the incidence of coronary heart disease. *Lancet* 1973; **i**: 333–39.

28 Morris JN, Everitt MG, Pollard R *et al.* Vigorous exercise in leisure time: protection against coronary heart disease. *Lancet* 1980; **ii**: 1207–10.

29 Morris JN, Clayton DG, Everitt MG *et al.* Exercise in leisure time: coronary attacks and death rates. *Br Heart J* 1990; **63**: 325–34.

30 Paffenbarger RS, Hale WE. Work activity and coronary heart mortality. *N Engl J Med* 1975; **292**: 545–50. Paffenbarger RS, Laughlin ME, Gima AS, Black RA. Work activity of longshoremen as related to death from coronary heart disease and stroke. *N Engl J Med* 1970; **282**: 1109–14.

31 Paffenbarger RS, Wing AL, Hyde RT. Physical activity as an index of heart attack risk in college alumni. *Am J Epidemiol* 1978; **108**: 161–75.

32 Paffenbarger RS, Hyde RT, Wing AL, Hseih CC. Physical activity, all cause mortality, and longevity of college alumni. *N Engl J Med* 1986; **314**: 605–13.

33 Kannel WB, Belanger A, D'Agostino R, Israel I. Physical activity and physical demand on the job and risk of cardiovascular disease and death: The Framingham Study. *Am Heart J* 1986; **112**: 820–25.

34 Kaplan GA, Strawbridge WJ, Cohen RD, Hungerford LR. Natural history of leisure-time physical activity and its correlates: Associations with mortality from all causes and cardiovascular disease over 28 years. *Am J Epidemiol* 1996; **144**: 793–7.

35 Pwell KE, Thompson PD, Casperson CJ, KEndricks JS. Physical activity and the incidence of coronary heart disease. *Annu Rev Publ Health* 1987; **8**: 253–87.

36 Hill AB. The environment and disease: association or causation. *Proc R Soc Med* 1965; **68**: 295–300.

37 Berlin JA, Colditz A. A meta-analysis of physical activity in the prevention of coronary heart disease. *Am J Epidemiol* 1990; **132**: 612–27.

38 Magnus K, Matroos A, Strackee J. Walking, cycling or gardening with or without seasonal interpretation in relation to acute coronary events. *Am J Epidemiol* 1979; **110**: 724–33.

39 Shapiro S, Weinblaff E, Franck CW *et al.* Incidence of coronary heart disease in population insured for medical care (HIP); myocardial infarction, angina pectoris and possible myocardial infarction. *Am J Publ Health* 1969: **59** (suppl 2): 1–101.

40 Slattery ML, Jacobs DR, Nichaman MZ. Leisure time physical activity and coronary heart disease death: The US Railroad Study. *Circulation* 1989; **79**: 304–11.

41 Blair SN, Kohl HW, Paffenbarger RS *et al.* Physical fitness and all cause mortality: A prospective study of healthy men and women. *JAMA* 1989; **262**: 2395–401.

42 Ekelund LG, Haskell WL, Johnson JL *et al.* Physical fitness as a predictor of cardiovascular mortality in asymptomatic North American men. The Lipids Research Clinics Mortality follow up study. *N Engl J Med* 1988; **319**, 1379–84.

43 Blair SN, Kohl HW, Gordon NF, Paffenbarger RS. How much physical activity is good for health? *Annu Rev Publ Health* 1992; **13**: 99–126.

44 A collection of physical activity questionnaires for health related research. Supplement to *Med Sci Sports Exer* 1997; **29**(6).

45 Sobolski J, Kornitzer M, de Backer G *et al.* Protection against heart disease in the Belgian Physical Fitness study: physical fitness rather than physical activity. *Am J Epidemiol* 1987; **125**: 601–10.

46 Blair SN, Kohl HW, Barlow CE *et al.* Physical fitness and all cause mortality. *JAMA* 1995; **273**: 1093–8.

47 Sandvik L, Erikssen J, Thaulow E *et al.* Physical fitness as a predictor of mortality among healthy middle aged Norwegian men. *N Engl J Med* 1993; **328**: 353–8.

48 Peters RK, Cady LD, Bischoff DP *et al.* Physical fitness and subsequent myocardial infarction in healthy workers. *JAMA* 1983; **249**: 3052–6.

49 Blair SN, Kampert JB, Kohl HW *et al.* Influences of cardiorespiratory fitness and other precursors on cardiovascular disease and all cause mortality in men and women. *JAMA* 1996; **276**: 205–10.

50 Kushi LH, Fee RM, Folsom AR, *et al.* Physical activity and mortality in postmenopausal women. *JAMA* 1997: **277**: 1287–92.

51 Superko HR. Exercise training, serum lipids, and lipoprotein particles: is there a change threshold? *Med Sci Sports Exer* 1991; **23**: 677–85.

52 MacAuley D, McCrum EE, Stott G, *et al.* Physical activity, physical fitness, lipids, apolipoproteins, and Lp(a) in the Northern Ireland Health and Activity Survey. *Med Sci Sports Exer* 1996; **28**: 720–37.

53 Durstine JL, Haskell WL. Effects of exercise training on plasma lipids and lipoproteins. In *Exercise and Sports Science Reviews* (JO Holloszy (Ed)). Willis and Wilkins, Baltimore, 1994: 477–521.

54 Montoye HJ, Mentzer HL, Keller JB. Habitual activity and blood pressure. *Med Sci Sports Exer* 1972; **4**: 175–181.

55 Gordon NF, Scott CB, Wilkinson WJ, Duncan JJ, Blair SN. Exercise and mild essential hypertension. Recommendations for adults. *Sports Med* 1990; **10**: 390–404.

56 Paffenbarger RS, Hyde RT, Wing AL, Hsieh CC. Physical activity and hypertension: An epidemiological review. *Ann Med* 1991; **23**: 319–27.

57 Reaven PD, Barrett-Connor E, Edelstein S. Relationship between leisure time physical activity and blood pressure in older women. *Circulation* 1991; **83**: 559–65.

58 Leon AS, Connett J, Jacobs DR, Rauramaa R. Leisure time physical activity levels and the risk of coronary heart disease and death. The Multiple Risk Factor Intervention Trial. *JAMA* 1987; **258**: 2388–95.

59 Shaper AG, Wannamethee G. Physical activity and ischaemic heart disease in middle aged British men. *Br Heart J* 1991; **66**: 384–94.

60 Hagberg JM. Exercise, fitness and hypertension. In *Exercise, Fitness and Health. A Consensus of Current Knowledge.* (Bouchard C, Shepherd RJ, Stephens T, Sutton J, MacPherson B Eds) Human Kinetics, Champaign IL, 1988: 455–66.

61 Blair SN, Goodyear NN, Gibbons LW, Cooper KH. Physical fitness and incidence of hypertension in healthy normotensive men and women. *JAMA* 1984; **252**: 487–90.

62 Stamler R, Stamler J, Gosch FC. The primary prevention of hypertension by nutritional–hygienic means: Final report of randomised clinical trial. *JAMA* 1989; **262**: 1801–807.

63 Van Baak MA. Exercise and hypertension: facts and uncertainties. *Br J Sports Med* 1988: **32**: 6–10.

64 Kannel WB, Wolf PA, Castelli WP, D'Agostimo RB. Fibrinogen and risk of cardiovascular disease. The Framingham Study. *JAMA* 1987; **258**: 1183.

65 Wilhelmsen L, Svardsudd K, Korsan-Bengtson K *et al.* Fibrinogen as a risk factor for stroke and myocardial infarction. *N Engl J Med* 1984; **311**: 501.

66 Rosengren A, Wilhelmsen L, Welin T *et al.* Social influences and cardiovascular risk factors as determinants of plasma fibrinogen concentration in a general population sample of middle aged men. *BMJ* 1990; **300**: 634–8.

67 Elwood PC, Yarnell JWG, Pickering J *et al.* Exercise, fibrinogen, and other risk factors for ischaemic heart disease: Caerphilly Prospective Heart Disease Study. *Br Heart J* 1993; **69**: 183–7.

68 Lee AJ, Smith WCS, Lowe GDO, Tunstall-Pedoe H. Plasma fibrinogen and coronary risk factors: The Scottish Heart Health Study *J Clin Epidemiol* 1990; **9**: 913–9.

69 Connelly JB, Cooper JA, Meade TW. Strenuous exercise, plasma fibrinogen, and factor VII activity. *Br Heart J* 1992; **67**: 351–4.

70 Folson AR, Wu KK, Davis CE *et al.* Population correlates of plasma fibrinogen and factor VII, putative cardiovascular risk factors. *Atherosclerosis* 1991: **91**: 191–205.

71 Ernst E. Regular exercise reduces fibrinogen levels: a review of longitudinal studies. *Br J Sports Med* 1993; **27**: 175–6.

72 Meade TW, Mellows S, Brozovic M *et al.* Haemostatic function and ischaemic heart disease: principal results of the Northwick Park Heart Study. *Lancet* 1986; **2**: 533.

73 DeBusk RF, Stenestrand, Sheehan M, Haskell WL. Training effects of long versus short bouts of exercise in healthy subjects. *Am J Cardiol* 1990; **65**: 1010–13.

74 NIH Consensus Development panel on Physical Activity and Cardiovascular Health. *JAMA* 1996; **276**: 241–6.

75 MacAuley DA. Descriptive epidemiology of physical activity from a Northern Ireland perspective. *I J Med Sci* 1994; **163**: 228–33.

76 Allied Dunbar National Fitness Survey. *Activity and Health Research* 1992.

77 MacAuley D, McCrum EE, Stott G *et al. The Northern Ireland Health and Activity Survey Report.* Belfast, HMSO, 1994.

78 *Heartbeat Wales. Pulse of Wales*: preliminary report of the Welsh Heart Health Survey. Heartbeat Wales Report No 4. Cardiff: Health Promotion Authority for Wales, 1985.

79 *Heartbeat Wales. Recent Trends in Lifestyles in Wales.* Technical Report Number 24. Cardiff: Health Promotion Authority for Wales, 1992.

80 Tunstall-Pedoe H, Smith WC, Crombie IK, Tavendale R. Coronary risk factor and lifestyle variation across Scotland: results from the Scottish Heart Health Study. *Scot Med J* 1989; **34**: 556–60.
81 *General Household Survey*. HMSO, London, 1990.

3 Promoting activity

Most people recognise the benefits of exercise and the advantage of taking part in physical activity. Many people are active when they are young but their activity levels decrease as they get older. Some decide to become active again and find it difficult to restart but most others who have adopted a sedentary lifestyle have no particular interest in becoming active again. The mental process leading to participation in physical activity is complex but has been modelled in four phases: adoption, maintenance, relapse and resumption [1]. As primary care physicians this presents us with a number of challenges. Some general practitioners become involved in activity promotion, while others take a less proactive role and counsel only those in whom there is a clear indication or who seek help. Most focus on getting people started and introducing people to the possibility of exercise. Few are in a position to influence how people sustain their activity programme, to check if they continue their programme, or encourage them to start again, other than in the normal course of the consultation.

There have been a number of innovative programmes in the United Kingdom encouraging people to become active but there has been very little evaluation of these methods and there is little evidence of their effectiveness. Clearly there are benefits of activity, and most people accept the value of exercise in theory. The challenge is in getting people active and finding strategies to modify community levels of physical activity. A systematic review [2] of population strategies to improve participation in physical activity examined the evidence. They selected only high quality studies using randomised controlled trials and identified 11 trials, but none of these studies was based in the United Kingdom.

The most effective methods were those that were home based, of moderate intensity, involved walking and had regular follow up. In contrast to the emphasis on structured exercise programmes based at leisure centres with which we are most familiar in the United Kingdom, the most effective programmes encouraged moderate intensity exercise and the most successful were based on walking from home. This is good news because walking is popular and is not perceived as a 'sport'. Brisk walking is also in keeping with the advice from the Surgeon General in the United States which changed the public health message and now encourages that 'every adult should accumulate 30 minutes or more of moderate intensity physical activity on most, preferably all, days of the week'. Brisk walking is also seen as achievable by the majority of patients. There are no access problems and no special equipment required. Injuries are less likely and it is acceptable socially. Brisk walking may also improve fitness. The Allied Dunbar national fitness survey [3] in England and the Northern Ireland health and activity survey [4] found population fitness levels of such a low level that brisk walking would have a training effect even for some young people. This type of intervention is sustainable and research indicates that when home based walking is the basis of an exercise promotion scheme, people were still active two years later. Probably the most important feature identified in the review of physical activity schemes identified above was that regular follow-up of participants encouraged long-term participation. This key feature in maintaining adherence to a programme is relatively inexpensive and could be easily delegated to another health professional such as a practice nurse.

Many of the recent initiatives in encouraging physical activity in general practice have been variations of exercise prescription schemes. In these schemes, the GP or practice nurse encourages patients to attend an exercise scheme, usually based at a local leisure centre or exercise group. This type of scheme has not been shown to be effective. In general, few patients are referred, with some estimates of less than 1% of a GP list, and there have been few measures of outcome. Some of these schemes may be effective but there is little published evidence. Fox and colleagues [5] identified 157 existing and 35 planned exercise promotion schemes in England. There were two basic models: general practice based models and leisure centre based models. The leisure centre based models were generally mediated through an exercise prescription scheme or general practitioner referral. They found that there were increases in short-term fitness and activity and improvements in well-being. The main weakness was that these schemes did not have long-term funding and that they had not been rigorously evaluated. Overall, however, the results did give cause for optimism because those general practitioners who took part were enthusiastic, leisure centres were willing to take on the responsibility and patients enjoyed it. In contrast, however, not all general practitioners were interested and the programmes only reach a small proportion of patients on any general practitioner list. One major advantage of the general practice initiated scheme is that it can provide a whole person perspective and that exercise can be seen in the context of overall health. The evidence for the effectiveness and cost effectiveness of such schemes has not been fully evaluated. Until randomised controlled trials which evaluate the long-term effectiveness of such schemes are available we cannot be certain of their value and these trials must look at different types of exercise schemes applied to different populations.

Overall the effectiveness of this type of general practice referral or exercise prescription scheme has not been demonstrated conclusively. The available evidence suggests that this method is not effective and that a home based programme of moderate exercise (for which brisk walking is ideal) with long-term follow-up and support will be most effective.

General practitioners may also be concerned about medicolegal responsibility in the event of a mishap associated with patient participation in such a scheme. The evidence for the benefit of exercise is so overwhelming that doctors should positively encourage exercise. Indeed any who discourage participation in physical activity are giving advice contrary to the established medical evidence. Clearly, exercise encouragement is appropriate and in keeping with current medical practice. In normal practice one would not be expected to have specialist knowledge but to provide advice of the kind usually advised by general practitioners. This expectation is enshrined in the legal duty of care which is to provide a service of the standard expected to be reached by a responsible body of medical opinion, now known as the Bolam test [6].

The exercise prescription must, of course, be appropriate for the individual patient, bearing in mind that the general practitioner should be the person best equipped to judge the patient's level of fitness and general health. The doctor should also be able to counsel the patient as to the risks and hazards of such exercise. If the doctor refers the patient to someone else, such as a fitness instructor or leisure centre, then the doctor should take some steps to ensure that the person or organisation to whom they have referred is suitably qualified. If the doctor refers the patient to a practice employee, then the doctor has a responsibility to ensure that such staff are competent. An employee, perhaps a practice nurse, would expect to be covered against claims for damages by the practice, but the doctor cannot be held vicariously liable for fitness staff or those not employed by the doctor [7].

It is likely that the best overall strategy for getting people active will be a combination of many methods and with the help of many different agencies. This will include an individual strategy, group efforts, community programmes and population measures. It will also include people from a wide spectrum of different disciplines including both medicine and nursing, but also sports scientists, teachers and people in government departments, the leisure centres and industry. It will also include many different types of organisation from charities to government agencies crossing the spectrum of community activity from the Departments of Health and Social Services to Environment. A review [8] of the methods used to encourage people to exercise identified a number of important factors. In order to get people to exercise one must focus on a target population and identify the level of intervention, select a theoretical model for the intervention, include self efficacy as a component and have reasonable outcome expectations, consider motivation level of the target group and evaluate the results. When looking at the factors that influence how a health professional influences physical activity, the personal behaviour of the professional also affects the outcome [9].

Encouraging people to exercise

If exploring factors that encourage people to be active we must look first at the motivational factors. Research has shown that these factors differ between men and women. Research also demonstrates that, in most cases, people are aware of the benefits of exercise and consider exercise to be very important as a means of staying healthy. While people are aware of the health benefits and it features high on their list of reasons to exercise there are others factors which have little to do directly with health but which are much more related to the packaging of the exercise message. Both men and women feel that exercise can help one to feel in good shape physically. This is supported by a considerable research base showing that exercise can improve mood and well-being and even recent research suggesting that it can improve creativity [10]. Other factors ranked as important by both men and women include how exercise can help one to feel alert mentally. Clearly the physical and psychological health messages are getting across.

Men and women may have different reasons for exercise, but while both men and women believe that exercise helps one to feel in good shape physically and to improve or maintain health, women consider health to be the more important reason. It is arguable whether we should use this as the prime factor in motivating women or if we should look to using other more market friendly factors in promoting physical activity to women.

Men believe exercise is important to help them feel mentally alert and to get out of doors and they also believe that exercise is of value in gaining a sense of achievement. These are interesting factors in that they show a particularly male pattern of motivation. One of the most interesting factors in encouraging women to exercise is the concept of body image and women rate 'looking good' as one of the most important benefits of exercise.

It is clear that people have accepted the health message but there are many other factors that have relevance. In our leisure orientated population about 80% believe that having fun is key to a healthy lifestyle and just over two thirds of the population believe this can be achieved through exercise. Similarly, more than 80% believe that it is important to relax and forget about one's cares and just over half believe that this can be achieved through exercise.

Reasons for ceasing exercise participation

In competition with the exercise message and the many schemes promoting exercise, are many psychological and logistical barriers to participation which can partly explain why some people do not take up, or lose interest in, exercise programmes.

If we wish to encourage people to take more exercise then we really ought to look closely at these barriers and disincentives and try to reduce their influence. When asked why they have given up regular participation in sport or active recreation during their adult years people list a number of factors. Of those who give up exercise, the main factors listed are work, that they lost interest in the activity, or that they needed time to do other things. For women, child care and responsibility for the family are major factors and about 30% of women report that caring for children prevents their participation. These are important limits to participation. When we examine other factors that could influence participation we find other domestic and family factors such as marriage or a change in partner. Major barriers clearly do exist and is it insufficient merely to encourage people to become active. There must be cooperation across the leisure industry to make it easier for people to take part in exercise through provision of child care facilities and opportunities to exercise at times that are convenient, bearing in mind family and domestic responsibilities.

It is also important to be aware of the public perception of exercise. The way that exercise is marketed or promoted can greatly affect public willingness to participate. One of the major messages from recent research is that exercise and sport are not the same and are not necessarily interchangeable. The public perception that physical activity means sport may be one of the major psychological barriers to be overcome.

Including exercise into our current busy lifestyle is a major challenge. For most people it is difficult to fit in all the essential daily tasks and exercise is considered an optional extra. It is not surprising that lack of time is considered the greatest barrier of all to exercise and is the reason given by over one third of men and almost one half of all women.

Exercise prescription

Exercise prescription schemes have some merit in that they recognise the need to build inter-professional bridges between doctors and other community organisations. While success may be limited, these schemes highlight the need to ensure that we do not medicalise exercise. To promote exercise effectively there should be broad support from government departments and charitable organisations including health, education and the environment with links to after school centres, leisure centres etc.

The key questions are how we can get people active and keep them active. Our main intervention tool in general practice is, and has always been, either the prescription or the referral letter and new initiatives in general practice have tended to focus on this traditional model. The exercise prescription thus became the model for exercise intervention. Of a number of experiments with the exercise prescription schemes, few have had critical evaluation.

In some cases the exercise prescription scheme has worked as a result of an almost evangelical zeal on behalf of the protagonists. A doctor's suggestion to undertake an exercise programme is only the beginning and to be effective there must be multi-disciplinary support.

There are a number of psychological barriers. Initially we thought of motivation as a one-dimensional concept but with time we have begun to explore other psychological models, particularly the stages of change model [11]. In this model, those who are encouraged to exercise may change from a pre-contemplation to a contemplation phase and hence to an action stage. Moving through these stages of change requires facilitation at all stages but one can slip back at any time. Using this model, the exercise action then requires a sustained and facilitated psychological movement. This stage of change model has been validated [12] and used successfully in counselling sedentary people [13].

Combined with these psychological factors there are other more tangible barriers. Some of the more important can be classified into physical, emotional, motivational, time and availability. These barriers may include some injury or disability and this applies to 1 in 5 of the population with an age related increase. One may argue, of course, that exercise is of benefit to all, irrespective of their level of fitness or ability but it is also important to consider the physical limitations that people perceive. Poor health is also considered a barrier and in some studies up to 1 in 3 of those aged over 55 considered this to be a major barrier. Up to 30% of those over 55 years old consider themselves too old and about 1 in 4 consider themselves to be too fat.

Project PACE

PACE is an acronym for Physician-based Assessment and Counselling for Exercise [14]. This is a major North American project aimed at getting people active. It is issued by the Center for Disease Control in Atlanta and is evidence based. The PACE materials include a manual which contains all the up-to-date information pointing to the benefits of physical activity. There are various other resource materials and details on the three counselling protocols. It includes an assessment form which has two major components. The first is an attempt to establish the patient's stage of change. Depending on the stage of change there are three counselling programmes aimed at getting people active. The second is the Physical Activity Readiness Questionnaire (PAR-Q) which can be used to screen for potential health problems needing further assessment. There is an excellent algorithm indicating who should be allowed to exercise. It also includes a section dealing with responses to questions that patients may ask in broad terms about the who, what, how often, where, why and how. The project PACE manual is an excellent resource for those undertaking physical activity health promotion in primary care.

The PACE programme recommends the following key components of a physical activity programme:

- a warm-up period lasting 5–10 minutes which may include low intensity activity, stretching or calisthenics,
- an activity phase based on the acronym FITT (Frequency, Intensity, Type and Time), and
- a cool-down period for 5–10 minutes similar to the warm-up, but including activity such as walking or stretching.

Advice for patients includes the following.

- How to exercise: continuous exercise of the large muscle groups such as walking/jogging/swimming/cycling/dancing and similar activities.
- How often: the target is to exercise on most days of the week. For those who are unaccustomed to exercise a reasonable goal would be exercise twice each week. This may be gradually increased to exercise on three days per week.
- How hard: the target is moderate intensity. Moderate intensity is exercise which produces a heart rate of 50–70% of maximum heart rate. (Theoretical maximum is 220 minus ones age). At moderate intensity one should be able to carry on a conversation.
- How long: at least 20 minutes but up to 1 hour in duration depending on the intensity.

Exercise and heart disease

Many of the commonly prescribed drugs can alter the individual's response to exercise and must be identified in the pre-exercise medical history. Such medications include β-blockers, vasodilators, diuretics, digitalis and anti-arrhythmic agents. Each has the potential to affect the response to exercise and training and may affect both heart rate and or blood pressure. There may also be associated changes in the ECG response to exercise. These changes have implications for training, and in monitoring training as there may not be the expected cardiovascular changes during exercise.

Exercise should be integrated with other forms of lifestyle modification in general practice. There are often some misconceptions and some patients are under the misguided belief that by exercising they can counteract the adverse effects of smoking. Clearly this is not true. Those patients taking up exercise should also be advised on diet and to lose weight if obese. The appropriate diet is a high fibre/low fat diet and many now advise additional antioxidants. Epidemiological evidence suggests low-dose aspirin and perhaps low-dose alcohol in the older population. There is also evidence in favour of fish oil supplements and perhaps trace elements.

Cardiac rehabilitation

An exercise-based cardiac rehabilitation programme can help reduce cardiovascular mortality. There is evidence from several studies that exercise training significantly reduces mortality, with a reduction of up to 25% in those where other risk factors are also controlled. As well as a reduction in mortality there are improvements in the symptoms of ischaemic heart disease through reduced angina. The reduction in angina is probably due to reduced myocardial oxygen requirement through improved fitness. There is also improvement in functional fitness independent of objective measures of improvement in myocardial perfusion so that patients have increased exercise tolerance and functional capacity. There is proven benefit in patients with cardiac failure, even in the absence of objective improvements in cardiac function. Of course, local muscle fitness is also improved by conditioning exercise, which improves general functional fitness. In addition to the objective measures of function, there are also well recognised improvements in psychological well-being and quality of life.

The risk of death during these programmes is low. Those who are at greatest risk are those who have poor cardiac function at baseline and those who do not exercise regularly and frequently. There is the paradox, however, that those with the lowest baseline fitness level have the most to gain by physical activity.

Physical activity has been a part of cardiac rehabilitation programmes in hospital for some time. This was pioneered in North America, although it is becoming more a feature of UK practice.

There are, as yet, few opportunities in primary care although clearly the potential is there. One of the pioneers of this form of cardiac rehabilitation in the United Kingdom is Dr Hugh Bethell [15–17].

At first it seemed strange to encourage patients to exercise when they had proven coronary artery disease. It seemed even more unusual to exercise those who had had a myocardial infarction. However, exercise is now accepted as an integral part of cardiac rehabilitation. Using exercise to aid rehabilitation was first pioneered in Canada. These were ambitious programmes where one of the expected graduation achievements of the rehabilitation was for the patient to complete a marathon run. The effectiveness of exercise in rehabilitation has been well proven and is accepted as a valid and effective intervention.

The programme is based on regular low intensity exercise within controlled levels of intensity. In theory this could be part of a general practice intervention and indeed has been used by office based primary care physicians in the United States. There is evidence of benefits in reducing both cardiac mortality and morbidity where the main modifiable risk factors are hypertension, hypercholesterolaemia, smoking and physical inactivity. The heart responds to programmes of physical activity. There are macro- and micro-changes. There is an increase in end diastolic size and volume. There is an improvement in ventricular contraction and function. One of the particular benefits is improvement of the myocardium, making it less susceptible to ischaemia.

The preparticipation medical examination

It can be difficult to know what to include in a pre-exercise medical examination. In different sports there are factors associated with the sport or sporting environment which may make participation more hazardous for people with certain medical conditions. This is a basic model for a medical questionnaire and examination. It is not comprehensive and doctors may prioritise some aspects of a medical history depending on the sport or add additional criteria.

Medical examination checklist

Name:

Address:

Phone no. (work and home)

GP name and address:

Questionnaire

Family history of:

Death before the age of 50 years

Heart problems

High blood pressure

Stroke

Diabetes

Epilepsy

Asthma

Allergies

Arthritis

Other Conditions

Current health

I am aware or have been told I have problems with:

Vision/poor sight

Hearing

Teeth (any problems with toothache or wisdom teeth)

Nose/throat (any problems with tonsillitis or swollen glands)

Headaches

Dizziness/light headedness

Numbness/pins and needles

Fits/faints

Loss of memory

Have you ever been concussed?

Back pain

Breathing problems/cough/short of breath/wheeze/spit

Poor appetite/vomiting/problems with bowels diarrhoea/constipation/passing blood

Problems passing urine/pain/blood

Period problems (may be discussed in private)

Any other problems

In the past I have had problems with:

Earache

Toothache

Glandular fever/viral illness

Blood pressure

Lung problems/asthma/short of breath

Diabetes

Thyroid problem

Jaundice/hepatitis

Epilepsy

Blood problems such as anaemia/bruising/haemophilia

Hernia

Arthritis

Broken bones – specify

Knee problems

Neck problems

▶

Surgery to my joints or bones

Problems with abdomen/kidneys/spleen/liver

Skin problems

Any other serious illness

When I exercise I sometimes get light headed/dizzy/irregular heartbeat

I have problems with heat

In the past I have had problems with:

Head: concussion/unconscious/skull fracture

Neck injury

Chest injury

Shoulder/arm/hand

Hip

Knee

Ankle

Feet

Smoking

Alcohol

Medication

Vitamins/electrolytes

Inhalers etc

I wish to discuss the possibility that I may have taken a prohibited substance (either by accident or deliberately)

Physical examination

References

1 Sallis JF, Hovell MF. Determinants of exercise behaviour. *Exer Sport Sci Rev* 1990; **18**: 307–30.
2 Hillsdon M, Thorogood M. A systematic review of physical activity promotion strategies. *Br J Sports Med* 1996; **30**: 84–9.
3 Allied Dunbar National Fitness Survey. London, *HEA/Sports Council*, 1992.
4 MacAuley D, McCrum EE, Stott G et al. *The Northern Ireland Health and Activity Survey. Government Publications HMSO*, 1994.
5 Fox K, Biddle S, Edmunds L et al. Physical activity promotion through primary health care in England. *Br J Gen Prac* 1997; **47**: 367–9.
6 Bolam v Friern Hospital Management Committee. 1957 QBD BMLR 1,1.
7 Day AT. Exercising medical judgement. *Br J Sports Med* 1997; **31**: 267–8.
8 Dunn AL. Getting started – a review of physical activity adoption studies. *Br J Sports Med* 1996; **30**: 193–9.
9 McDowell N, McKenna J, Naylor PJ. Factors that influence practice nurses to promote physical activity. *Br J Sports Med* 1997; **31**: 308–13.
10 Steinberg H, Sykes EA, Moss T et al. Exercise enhances creativity independently of mood. *Br J Sports Med* 1997; **31**: 240–45.
11 Prochaska JO, DiClemente CC. In search of how people change: applications to addictive behaviour. *Am J Psychol* 1992; **47**: 1102–14.
12 Marcus B, Simkin L. The stages of exercise behaviour. *J Sports Med Phys Fitness* 1993; **33**: 83–8.
13 Buxton K, Wyse J, Mercer T. How applicable is the stages of change model to exercise behaviour: A review. *Health Educ J* 1996; **55**: 239–57.
14 *Project Pace. Physician based Assessment and Counselling for Exercise*. Physician Manual. Centers for Disease Control, Cardiovascular Health Branch, Atlanta, Georgia, 1992.
15 Bethell H. Post-infarction problems. *Practitioner* 1993. **237**: 925–8.
16 Horgan J, Bethell H, Carson P et al. Working party report on cardiac rehabilitation. *Br Heart J* 1992; **67**: 412–18.
17 Bethell H. Rehabilitation after a myocardial infarction. *Practitioner* 1989; **233**: 335–339.

4 Background physiology

Patients often say that they 'would like to get fit' and ask how they should begin. Patients like to know how much they should train and what type of exercise they should do. There is no easy answer to this question and it depends on the purpose of their training. People have different ambitions and expectations from exercise. Some simply exercise for the health benefits and in particular to optimise their cardiovascular health and reduce the risk of atherosclerotic heart disease. Others exercise to lose weight, to improve their appearance, or to improve their performance in sport and competition. For those who train to compete, advice on training will be even more specialised and will depend on the nature of the sport and their ambitions within that sport. To help answer these questions, it is useful to revise some of the background physiology.

Training

Training is simply a planned progressive increase in physical activity, so that adaptation to that activity leads to an improvement in performance. So, if we train to improve our running ability, we gradually increase the training load in distance and intensity. Similarly, if we wish to swim or cycle we practise the activity. If weight lifting is our sport, the principles are the same with a progressive increase in load with adaptation, but the nature of the training programme will be slightly different. Training is specific to the activity performed so that an improvement in running only comes with running, rowing with rowing etc. There are, however, two components to training for endurance sport. There is a central cardiovascular training effect (which is common to all endurance sports) and there is local muscle adaptation (which is sports–specific). This sport-specific adaptation is also specific to the speed and duration of the activity, so that sprint and endurance training are different.

Physical activity and training have an effect on many parts of the body. There is both local muscle and central cardiac adaptation, but there is also adaptation of bones, joints and alterations to other parameters including cardiovascular risk factors such as blood pressure and lipids. The cardiac adaptations are probably the best known.

Changes in training include an increase in the size and efficiency of the heart. There is left ventricular hypertrophy but there is also an increase in the end diastolic volume and a general improvement in ventricular performance and contractile function giving improved efficiency. This leads to an increase in stroke volume and reduction in resting heart rate. Investigations show an increase in the R wave on electrocardiography and an increase in left ventricular wall measurement on echocardiography.

There is local muscle adaptation which occurs at both a macro- and microscopic level. There is hypertrophy of those muscle groups used in exercise and this is combined with improvements in the capillary circulation. There are intracellular changes with an increase in muscle enzymes and concentration of mitochondria. Different types of training encourage different adaptation. Heavy weight, low repetition, strength training encourages more muscle hypertrophy, while endurance training has more influence on microvasculature, enzymes and mitochondria. Differential changes occur at cellular level depending on the type of training and different types of muscle cells: some are more suitable for endurance and others for sprinting. Training selectively stimulates these different cells.

Metabolic changes occur with increase in bone deposition, changes in energy metabolism leading to more efficient transport of glucose, changes in iron metabolism and production of haemoglobin. There are changes in the ability to adapt to heat through sweating and minor changes in the lungs.

Types of training

Different types of training have different effects, and the same training can affect individuals differently. Training can modify genetic potential but this genetic potential is the main limiting factor. Some are born to be distance runners and some to be Sumo wrestlers.

Components of performance

Training can be broken down into a number of components, illustrated in the box below. Each different sport or activity will have a training mix determined by the nature of the sport.

Training: summary

Strength
Strength is associated with muscle bulk. It is developed using low repetitions of heavy weights. Strength is developed in the direction and speed of movement of the sport. It is associated with type 2, fast twitch muscle fibres.

Speed
Speed is dictated by the speed of muscle contraction. It is also associated with type 2, fast twitch muscle fibres, and can be related to muscle elastic component.

Stamina
Stamina or muscle endurance is determined by the ability to supply the muscles with sufficient oxygen to allow the muscles to perform for a period of time. Aerobic capacity is the term used most often in the context of endurance sport. It is defined by the ability to pick up oxygen from the lungs, transport it through the blood, supply it to the individual muscle cells and use it within the cells.

Skill
This is what we describe as natural talent, and eye for the ball and good hand–eye coordination. It is not so much a physiological parameter as a natural attribute. Some features such as spatial awareness and peripheral vision have some physiological background but for the most part these attributes cannot be measured using quantitative methods. In some people ball skills seem to be associated with left handedness. Some sports require skills that are actually repetitive movements of a simple task within very close limits, for example in rowing or gymnastics.

Spirit (psychology)
Recently qualitative methods have helped unravel the psychological factors associated with motivation. It is difficult to measure and train these attributes but there are some patterns such as the inverted U of the personality profile. The classic arousal performance curve has been used to illustrate the psychological relationship with performance, but this has now been superceded.

The main components are strength, speed, stamina (endurance), skill and spirit (psychology). Each of these parameters can be modified by training but each individual and each component responds differently to different stimuli. These five key components of fitness all have some genetic and/or familial background. It is possible to train each component to produce optimal performance although for the most part performance is determined by the genetic template. It is, however, possible to measure some physical components that can predict performance.

Factors in performance

Physiological tests can give an objective measure of fitness which can help predict performance. For example, muscle fibre type can offer some insight into a preference for endurance or sprinting. In sprinting the muscles contract very fast for a short period of time and this is associated with type 1 muscle fibres. Endurance capacity is associated with type 2. These muscle fibre types cannot be changed, so genetics determine that one is born with an affinity for one particular type of exercise. There is however some aerobic trainability associated with type 2b, but essentially one's ability to sprint or in endurance sport is determined genetically. A muscle biopsy gives some indication of potential but unfortunately, while there are statistical associations with performance, predictions are a little more difficult. For example, biopsies in different muscle groups and at different levels within the muscle may give different readings. In addition, one cannot predict how fast, a fast twitch predominant athlete will be.

It would be incorrect to think that sport can be neatly divided into sprinting and endurance events. The duration of exercise dictates which component contributes most to performance, but it is a continuum with contributions from both aerobic and anaerobic metabolism to every distance. When we use the terms aerobic and anaerobic we describe methods of energy production to supply muscle activity. Energy for immediate, very short duration activity, is supplied by intramuscular ATP and creatine phosphate. Intramuscular glycogen can be broken down with lactate production extending this to about 30 seconds. Sprinting or short duration activity that extends beyond a few seconds requires energy from another source. For this activity energy is supplied from breakdown of glycogen, in the absence of oxygen. This is an inefficient energy supply which produces lactate as a waste product, and lactate accumulation limits the duration of this type of activity. Aerobic activity is much more efficient with the breakdown of glycogen in the presence of oxygen. The waste products of this energy supply are carbon dioxide (CO_2) and water (H_2O). This energy supply is limited by the glycogen store which lasts only about 2 hours. Fat may be broken down as a slow energy supply but this metabolic pathway is rather slower and is only suitable for long duration low intensity activity.

Energy and metabolism

In aerobic metabolism glycogen is broken down to produce 39 moles of ATP from 180 g glycogen. The waste products, which are water (H_2O) and carbon dioxide (CO_2), cause no problems as they are transported in the bloodstream. The limiting factors are the supply of glycogen and oxygen. Glycogen is the energy substrate for aerobic exercise and it is this substrate availability which is one of the major determining factors in performance [1]. Glycogen supply depends on glycogen stores in the muscle and the liver. There is a relatively small supply of glycogen in the muscle cell but together the muscles and liver can store about 1800 kcal. The total storage capacity is sufficient for about 2 hours of aerobic exercise.

Additional metabolism is through breakdown of fat. In order to increase the availability of energy substrate athletes have tried to supplement the energy supply during exercise through consuming carbohydrate in solid or liquid, and to increase the glycogen storage by dietary manipulation. Such methods have had some success and are discussed later. There is no theoretical limit to oxygen availability in the air, but aerobic metabolism depends on providing an adequate supply of oxygen to the muscle cell. Training is one means of increasing oxygen supply through improvements in cardiorespiratory and local muscle endurance.

Sporting patients who are involved in endurance sports will be familiar with these concepts and will know about oxygen uptake and glycogen supply and storage. Some folk descriptions graphically illustrate the limitations of glycogen storage. Marathon runners describe 'hitting the wall' while cyclists may call it 'the knock' or 'the bonk'. These are the athletes' interpretation of what happens when they run out of fuel. In marathon running, when a runner has completed about 2 hours of the race, their muscles reach the end of the energy supply. This may occur between 18 and 22 miles, depending on their speed and when the energy supply is exhausted they feel as if they cannot run another step. This fatigue may be reduced by consuming carbohydrate but eating and drinking while running is difficult. The elite marathon runner is usually unaware of 'the wall'. They complete the marathon in little over two hours but, in addition, due to their long-term training the body has adapted and part of their energy needs are supplied through fat metabolism. For the leisure runner who takes much longer than two hours, the problems may be compounded. As they run out of energy substrate, the muscles cannot work as well, they do not produce as much heat, and are not only exhausted but with inadequate heat production, can become cold. Cyclists are also familiar with this problem, as their training and racing is often in excess of 2–3 hours. For this reason they constantly refuel, using either solid or liquid carbohydrate. It is much easier to consume and digest food while cycling as the body weight is supported.

Glycogen is not a major limiting factor in anaerobic sport where energy is produced using a shorter circuit of the Krebs cycle without oxygen. From a metabolic perspective this energy pathway is inefficient producing only 3 moles of ATP for 180 g of glycogen and the major limiting factor is the production of lactic acid. Lactic acid builds up in the cell inhibiting activity which the athlete feels as pain and stiffness in the muscles. This is the energy pathway used in sprints such as in the 100 m, 200 m and in team games. Usually there is an opportunity to recover and metabolise the lactic acid production after a major exertion.

Energy is also available from oxidation of fatty acids. This type of energy production is usually only of value in sustained low level exercise. More highly trained endurance athletes tend to be able to make more use of this energy source and for a given workload the endurance athlete can derive a greater proportion of energy from fatty acid metabolism. Caffeine was found to encourage an increase in fatty acid metabolism, and protection of glycogen stores, so there is some evidence of a beneficial effect on endurance sport.

Glycogen loading

There is scientific evidence to demonstrate a correlation between initial muscle glycogen and ability to maintain endurance work at 75% of maximum. Researchers focused on methods of increasing glycogen stores and found what is commonly known as the carbohydrate loading or glycogen boosting diet. Using this dietary regime, the athlete trains very hard for a few days on a low carbohydrate diet thus depleting glycogen stores. This makes the cells hungry for fuel. The athlete then eats a high carbohydrate diet, while training very lightly, and this should lead to supercompensation with greater than normal stores of glycogen. More recently athletes have begun to appreciate that the glycogen depletion phase may not be absolutely necessary as many are training in a state of constant energy deficit and in the period before competition it may be sufficient to taper training and increase consumption of a high carbohydrate diet.

Sport-specific training

Training is specific in that training improves performance best in the modalities in which one trains. Local muscle training is specific so that if one runs as training this will improve running performance, but not necessarily cycling performance. If one runs slowly this improves ones ability to run slowly but not in sprinting. A practical illustration is in the training of field sports. These sports are played as intermittent bursts of high intensity activity so that the ideal training is through sport-specific training. Encouraging players to train for endurance by running 10 circuits of the pitch simply makes them better able to run slowly and not more effective in play. When advising athletes on training it is important to emphasis the sport-specific nature of training and encourage them to tailor training towards their particular event. Sport-specific training can present other problems, in that endurance training can be boring and constant repetitive movements can cause overuse injuries. Thus a training programme must be specific, but varied. Putting together a training programme which is stimulating, exciting and enjoyable is the art of coaching. Simply based on science, training can become monotonous.

Aerobic exercise

The term aerobics is well known to us all. It was coined by Dr Ken Cooper, an American physiologist, to describe the rhythmic continuous form of exercise at a submaximal cardiovascular load. Cooper has become synonymous with this type of exercise, so much so that in some countries aerobic exercise is known as 'Cooperobics'. Examples of aerobic exercise include running, swimming and cycling. The term has evolved to include gym-based dance and exercise routines, which are only truly aerobic if they too exert a continuous submaximal cardiovascular load.

Aerobic exercise more accurately describes exercise of an intensity at which the body can supply sufficient oxygen for the muscles to metabolise glycogen in the most efficient way. The limiting factors in maintaining oxygen supply as the exercise intensity increases, are cardiac and the local muscle. Aerobic training aims to improve the ability of the body to transport oxygen to the muscles and to improve the ability of the muscles to use this oxygen.

Measuring fitness

The best method of measuring fitness is to measure performance in the event. This is the ultimate test, but we can use proxy measures of fitness which can help measure objectively the various components of fitness that make up performance. Some components of fitness are more easily measured than others; we are able to measure many parameters of endurance fitness. The efficiency of the muscle cell in using oxygen is what determines performance. Ideally we should measure the quantity of oxygen at cellular level. This is not possible. It is possible to measure the oxygen that reaches each individual muscle by measuring the oxygen in the artery leading to, and the vein leaving, the muscle. This is theoretically possible but very invasive. We can, however, measure all the oxygen that an athlete uses by measuring the oxygen inspired and expired, on the assumption that almost all the oxygen is used for muscle activity. If we exercise the athlete on a treadmill, we can then measure the quantity of oxygen used at different running speeds. Likewise, if we exercise a rower on a rowing ergometer or cyclist on a cycle ergometer we can get an accurate record of oxygen uptake at each workload. If we exercise an athlete on an ergometer, treadmill, cycle or rowing machine, and increase the workload in progressive increments we come to a point where the athlete is unable to increase their oxygen intake to meet the exercise demands. Although they can continue to exercise for a short period, and may even manage another increase in workload, they have reached their maximum oxygen uptake capacity, otherwise known as VO_2 max. When one reaches VO_2 max, the only way to increase the workload is by anaerobic metabolism, which generates lactate, and is ultimately the limiting factor. There is no simple switch between aerobic and anaerobic metabolism, and at VO_2 max the muscles are already producing lactic acid. Clearly one cannot exercise at the intensity equal to VO_2 max for long and performance in endurance is determined by the metabolism at submaximal level and the ability to recycle or tolerate lactate (see Figure 4.1). In sports where surges and sprints occur, such as cycling and some track races, this ability to recover from high intensity bursts on a background of high intensity aerobic exercise is a critical skill. Maximum oxygen uptake capacity is critical in aerobic exercise and has been used as an important measure of endurance fitness.

Measuring VO_2 max

Measuring VO_2 max is relatively simple and is performed frequently in the exercise physiology lab. There are two key pieces of equipment. An apparatus for measuring oxygen uptake, which simply measures the gas concentrations in inspired and expired air, and an ergometer which mimics closely the actual sport and where workload can be measured. A runner may use a treadmill and for other sports very sophisticated sport-specific ergometers are now available. Rowing ergometers mimic closely the workload in a boat, cyclists can now use their own cycles on quality ergometers and even swimmers use swimming flumes and measure oxygen uptake at different water speeds. It is essential to measure oxygen uptake using an exercise modality that is as close as possible to the sport itself. This is because training has developed such specific fitness that muscles are most efficient in the very specific modalities of the exercise itself and it is muscle efficiency in these exact movements at cellular level that determines fitness.

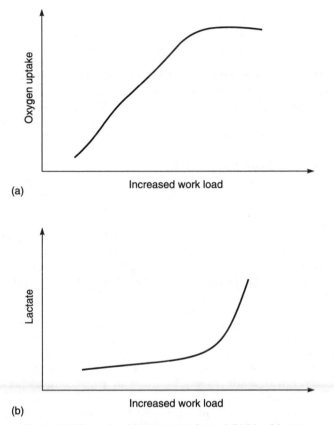

(a)

(b)

Figure 4.1 Measuring (a) oxygen intake and (b) blood lactate.

Lactic acid

Athletes may know their VO_2 max and will be able to discuss the relative merits of their own measurements. Maximal oxygen uptake capacity is to a great extent genetically determined and can only be improved by about 25% from sedentary by intensive training. It is not the maximum figure that is critical for performance, however, but the ability to perform at sub-maximal levels. Most training is directed towards improving one's performance at submaximal levels and increasing the proportion of VO_2 max at which one can compete. Submaximal thresholds may, therefore, be more important for performance. These include the point of onset of blood lactate (OBLA) as it is the ability to tolerate lactate that determines how long one can compete at submaximal level.

When exercise intensity increases we produce lactic acid. Some physiologists believe that the lactate–pyruvate ratio is a better estimate of aerobic status. However, when lactate is produced it is metabolised with the production of CO_2 and there is a related increase in CO_2 in expired air. So one of the first changes to be seen is an increase in CO_2 level. This indicates an increase in the level of exercise intensity. Usually this is at about 50% of maximum level.

Lactate increases with exercise intensity and reaches a level at which exercise can be sustained without a rapid increase. This is the maximum level of sustainable lactate and is usually at a level of about 4–5 mmol. In some athletes the level of sustainable exercise can as high as 8 mmol and very occasionally higher. These are exceptional athletes. At this level of activity, however, glycogen is metabolised anaerobically with production of CO_2 and exercise is metabolically inefficient. At this higher intensity level there is an increase in lactate, increase in acidity and a reduction in pH.

Training for endurance sport is aimed at improving athletic performance, but improvement can be measured by changes in these laboratory variables. Thus training for endurance sport has a number of different components. Long slow distance work aims to improve the aerobic metabolism of the local muscle. At a cellular level this leads to an increase in muscle mitochondria, increases in muscle enzyme production and increases in local muscle capillaries. High intensity work, including interval training, is aimed towards improving the ability of the body to tolerate submaximal lactate levels by exercising above race pace and producing a higher level of lactate than would normally be produced. True Fartlek training is a mixture of intensity and duration of bursts which aids the ability to cope with different types of change in pace and even endurance runners need some sprint training for speed. The science of training suggests the intensity of training required for each individual component, while the art of training is in knowing how much of each the athlete can manage without getting fatigued, bored or stale.

References

1 Hultman E, Greenhaf PL. Food stores and energy reserves. In: *Endurance in Sport* (Shepherd RJ, Astrand PO, Eds) Blackwell Science, Oxford, 1992.

5 Exercise for older people

Exercise maintains function and fitness with increasing age. It helps maintain strength, flexibility and endurance so we can undertake all the normal tasks of daily living as we become older. Exercise in the older person is of more benefit to quality of life than duration, by improving function, reducing falls, minimising ill health, and promoting independence. Exercise in the older person is about maintaining health and independence as long as possible. It is not so much about the length of life alone but about maintaining health as long as possible within one's lifetime [1]. It is the compression of morbidity into the latter years. The two key fitness components that deteriorate as we become older are strength and endurance, but we should not think of these in a sporting context, exercise performance is not the critical factor. The main focus of exercise in the older person is on fitness for life and maintaining quality of life. One of the early classic studies [2] showed how a progressive resistance exercise programme, even in a very elderly population, could increase and maintain faculties necessary for daily living.

Women live seven or eight years longer than men on average, so it is arguably more important to maintain strength and mobility in older women. Strength and power decrease with age, but the training effect of exercise can help minimise this age-related deterioration. Exercise improves the strength and function of muscle but may also modify tendons and ligaments [3] and influence the structure of bone. Inactivity leads to atrophy and although there is always an age-dependent loss of muscle bulk and strength [4] those who continue to exercise do not have the same deterioration in muscle function as controls [5]. Exercise and training should, therefore, be an integral part of the lifestyle of the elderly.

Age-related changes

With the age-related deterioration of muscle function, there is considerable loss of muscle mass, and thus loss of strength, so that 20–40% of total muscle mass is lost by the age of 80 years. Most of this loss occurs after the age of 60, with a 15% loss per decade after the age of 60 years [6]. Atrophy leads to loss of muscle bulk and, at cellular level, both a reduction of the number of muscle cells and deterioration in muscle fibres. Muscles become less effective, the muscle tissue is more difficult to stimulate, fatigues more easily and is metabolically less efficient. There is also a reduction in flexibility and muscle elasticity with increased likelihood of muscle injury. With age-related muscle atrophy there is a reduction in the lean body mass and one would expect an overall weight loss, but this does not always happen and the muscle mass may be replaced by fat. Exercise can have an additional effect, not just in maintenance of muscle mass, but in reducing the age-related increase in body fat that occurs with an increasingly sedentary lifestyle.

Recent research has investigated how much of this deterioration is as an inevitable result of ageing, or if it is due to lack of use. There is now considerable evidence to show that some age-related changes can be reversed by physical activity including physical training. Research demonstrates how regular sustained resistance exercise can help maintain strength and local muscle endurance. Performing a variety of exercises helps maintain overall flexibility and the range of muscle movement. This improved muscle function helps people retain their local muscle strength and endurance so they cope better with the tasks of daily living.

Cardiorespiratory fitness declines with age and there is a reduction in maximum oxygen uptake capacity by about 10% each decade. This is due to changes both in cardiovascular and local muscle fitness. The age-related changes in heart rate are used in the estimation of theoretical maximum heart rate which is 200 – age. There is also a deterioration in respiratory function with a decrease in forced vital capacity (FVC). Bone density reduces, especially in postmenopausal women.

Illness and medication

Exercise is not contraindicated in cardiac disease, as there are clear benefits in increasing exercise tolerance. Those with stable heart or respiratory disease may exercise but should use their nitrates or respiratory stimulants before exercise as appropriate; β-blockers can increase fatigue and reduce the heart rate response to exercise so that those who use β-blockers should monitor exercise intensity using perceived exertion rather than heart rate. Diuretics affect fluid and electrolyte balance and their use must be taken into consideration, especially if exercising in the heat. Postural hypotension can occur in patients taking some antihypertensive agents. Other medications may also affect exercise. Some antidepressants can increase drowsiness, increase sweating and reduce the sensation of thirst. Care should be taken by diabetics to monitor blood glucose and those who inject insulin should be careful about injection sites.

Physical activity has always been a major component of rehabilitation in patients with stroke. Those with arthritis should participate only in low impact exercise within the comfortable range of movement. Arthritis is usually accompanied by wasting of the adjacent muscle groups so that exercise can be of benefit by improving strength, tone, coordination and flexibility. Exercise is not appropriate, however, when a joint is acutely inflamed. Stiffness is usually greatest in the morning so exercise is best in the evening or after analgesia. Those with severe arthritis may be unable to undertake weightbearing activity but can still benefit from flexibility exercises or weight supported exercise such as swimming.

A moderate resistance exercise programme is also safe even in those who have established medical conditions such as diabetes, heart disease, hypertension, stroke and osteoporosis. For resistance exercise, most of which is non-weight-bearing, arthritis is not a contraindication. And where there is muscle wasting associated with arthritis, resistance exercise may be particularly useful.

Types of exercise for the older patient

Exercise does not just include jogging or working out at the gym but includes all the normal physical tasks that we undertake each day. Training may be planned with set objectives and a specific exercise routine, but many of the benefits can also be achieved by simply increasing the physical work in our daily lives or substituting a more physical alternative for some of the tasks for which we now use machines. Exercise can be integrated into normal daily life by taking the stairs rather than the lift, using a brush rather than the vacuum cleaner, walking rather than taking the car. There are opportunities for exercise in almost every ordinary daily task and one does not have to go to the gym. An older person can perform a very adequate routine at home using only the furniture and normal household equipment.

The ideal exercise programme would include both types of exercise: endurance training which focuses on cardiovascular fitness and resistance training which improves muscle strength. The term 'endurance training' is rather off-putting for the older patient, but this simply describes any continuous rhythmic exercise which raises the heart rate and keeps the muscles moving for a sustained period of time. It includes walking, cycling and swimming, but can equally include a sustained period of time spent brushing leaves, cutting the grass, or raking flowerbeds. Training in this manner improves the ability of the body to undertake this sustained type of exercise more easily in the future.

Resistance training is directed mostly at the maintenance and improvement of muscle strength. It may, of course, be formalised by doing specific exercises but not necessarily so. An ideal programme would include both endurance and resistance exercise but resistance training may be more important with increasing years. Before advising an older person to exercise, however, it is important to ensure that they are physically fit enough to undertake the exercise programme.

Current fitness levels

A recent British survey [7] which measured muscle strength and power, used measurements chosen to represent tasks appropriate to daily living. For example, the quadriceps strength was measured because of its importance in walking, cycling, running, climbing stairs and in changing posture, for example as in rising from a chair. Hand grip strength was chosen because of its importance in many tasks of daily living such as opening containers, holding, and carrying objects, and manipulating tools. Isometric knee extensor strength is an important functional parameter associated with movements such as getting out of a chair. For the purposes of establishing the proportion of each group who had inadequate strength for daily living, this survey compared strength measurements to a number of thresholds. It was suggested that, on the assumption that the normal knee extensor strength corresponds to approximately 75% of body weight, that when peak knee extensor strength is less than the strength required to lift 50% of body weight it is difficult to support the full body weight when standing with both feet on the ground and with the knees at an angle of 90°. The lower limits for functional knee extensor strength was thus set at 50% of body weight. Overall 24%, about 20% of men and 40% of women, fell below this functional threshold for knee extensor strength. Knee extensor strength declines with age and mean knee extensor strength in women is 62% that of men. Knee extensor strength deteriorated with age so almost 40% of men and 60% of women in the age group 55–74 years fell below this threshold.

While knee extensor strength is needed for movements such as getting out of a chair and maintenance of posture in flexion, leg extensor power reflects the explosive movement needed when climbing stairs or jumping. Mean leg extensor power in men is about 370 Watts and in women it is 180 Watts. Mean leg extensor power in women is about one half of male leg extensor power and there is a deterioration in leg extensor power with age in both sexes. On the basis that the power required to climb stairs is at least 2 Watts per kg, this defines a useful functional threshold. Only 3% of men but almost 25% of women fell below the threshold. The proportion who fell below the threshold increased with age, a feature that may be of particular importance when considering falls and osteoporotic fractures in older women. With these low levels of strength and power, and with the additional decline with age, a significant proportion of the older population have considerable functional impairment

Arm strength is important to help pull oneself up onto a bus, and carry shopping, Forearm and grip strength is important in opening jars, and gripping household equipment. Shoulder strength is important in pushing and pulling. When we use hand grip strength as an index of upper limb strength we find that about 10% of women fall below a functional threshold for hand grip equivalent to the strength required to lift 20% of bodyweight. Flexibility is a further index of functional fitness to carry out the normal tasks of daily living. Mean shoulder abduction in men and women is about 145° but 6% of men and 9% of women fall below the functional threshold of 120°. These figures give us food for thought in that a significant proportion of the older population fall below thresholds for adequate strength and power.

Types of training

Resistance training will make the muscles stronger and make it easier to carry out the normal activities of daily life. For many older people, simply getting out of a chair is a major task. The muscle strength in the legs alone may not be enough and they may need to use their hands to help by pushing themselves up. Clearly it is important to maintain leg strength as we get older. Being inactive or of poor fitness is not a contraindication to this type of training and perhaps the greatest benefits are to be gained by those who are least fit. Age is no barrier and one of the outstanding pieces of research in this decade was that which showed that an exercise programme could help increase strength in the very elderly, even those over 90 years. In this research, exercise improved not only the size and strength of muscles, but the elderly people were more mobile and became more active [89]. Indeed, rather than advising the frail elderly to avoid exercise, it is this group who have most to gain in improving muscle strength and flexibility and for whom maintenance of functional independence and prevention of falls is most important. A further recent research study showed how exercise could also help reduce depression in the elderly. It is unclear if this is biological or cognitive. Clearly there are physical benefits associated with achievement in an exercise programme but irrespective of the mechanism of the reduction in depression, the physical and psychological benefits both add to the quality of life. Certainly there appears to be a benefit.

Assessing risks

In theory anyone over 40 years old who has not been previously physically active should consult their doctor before undertaking a training programme. For older people, there is an increasing risk, especially in the sedentary. The American College of Sports Medicine [10] recommends an exercise stress test for all those over the age of 60 years of age and all those who have a history of ischaemic heart disease, angina, diabetes or hypertension should have one. It may also be advisable in those who smoke. Those on medication should consult their doctor, in particular those taking medication for hypertension, diabetes or any heart condition.

Exercise increases blood pressure so those with hypertension should be well controlled before exercising. Similarly, exercise may provoke exercise-induced bronchospasm so asthma should be well controlled and medication used appropriately. Those with arthritis should perform non-impact exercise only within the comfortable range of movement.

It is often difficult to tailor advice for our older patients as there can be great variation in the level of fitness and state of health. Those who are more fit and active can continue with normal aerobic type activity and with conditioning exercises in the gym or activities around the home such as gardening, washing the car, DIY etc. But those who are less fit or active can also benefit. The Research Centre on Ageing at Tufts University in Boston has a particular interest in the training of older people. The following notes are based on some of the work carried out at this laboratory. These notes are written so that they can be photocopied and given to patients in the consulting room.

Exercise for older people

Conditioning exercise

Exercise can benefit almost everyone and there are few reasons why you should not do some exercises, but you should discuss your own personal health and general condition with your doctor before starting an exercise programme. Set aside some time for exercise, about 20 to 30 minutes on at least 3 days each week. If muscle strength is poor, then simple exercises using your own body weight are a useful beginning, but as strength improves, it may be necessary to use slightly more sophisticated exercises. Training is aimed not at improving strength and muscle size but to make muscles more efficient.

With improved strength you are less likely to injure yourself around the house. The muscles will be stronger so you will be less likely to fall, your ligaments will be stronger so your joints will be more stable, and your bones will become stronger, so less likely to break if you do fall.

Aerobic training

We do some aerobic exercise in all our daily activities, walking, climbing stairs, swimming, even doing work around the house, although we tend to do less of this type of activity as we become older. Aerobic training is easy and requires no special exercises or equipment. It simply means increasing the duration and intensity of normal activities. For example, set a target of walking to the news-agent's each day, perhaps swimming once per week, ballroom dancing or bowling. These are simple, easy activities that can be integrated into daily living with minimal change in your routine. Many sport and leisure centres have classes or activity sessions aimed specifically at older people where the exercise is graded, varied, and monitored according to age and level of fitness. Your target should be 30 minutes of this type of activity on most days of the week. Exercise should cause no distress so choosing the level is important. The target exercise intensity should be just below that which would make you breathless. For those who would prefer a more specific target, you may use heart rate to set targets and grade your exercise so that your heart rate is about 60% of your maximum, assuming that the maximum is 220 minus your age and that you are not taking any medication, such as β-blockers. If you have a medical condition which makes walking difficult, swimming may be an option, and for those who cannot swim, your local leisure centre may offer water aerobics for which it is not necessary to be able to swim. Better to cycle than jog, swim than aerobics etc. Some leisure centres provide exercise equipment such as rowing, cycling, stair walking and skiing machines. The secret, as you get older, is to exercise within your limits and to avoid high impact or painful activities. It is best to start modestly and continue, rather than exercise vigorously and stop early.

Exercises for the older person

These are some basic exercises for those who cannot get out of the house or who do not wish to go to a leisure centre or sports club. These following exercises are aimed at those who are oldest and will gain most.

Leg exercises:

1. Sit on a hard high back chair, raise your leg slowly to the horizontal and then lower your leg again slowly. Do this ten times and then repeat it with the other leg. Sit on a straight high back chair so that the thigh is horizontal.
2. Stand up slowly from the sitting position and then sit down again slowly. Do this exercise ten times. Do this exercise slowly and try not to use your arms.

Shoulder exercises:

1. Lift one arm slowly above the head ten times. Repeat the exercise using the other arm. Then repeat the exercise using both arms.
2. When you can do this with ease, you may add some weights. You could use some light hand weights, but if you are careful you can use simple household goods such as a bag of dried peas for example. Use the same weight in each hand.

Forearm and hand:

1. Bend the arm slowly at the elbow ten times. Repeat with the other arm.
2. You can increase the resistant used in this exercise using simple household items. For example, use an orange as a weight. Hold the forearm out horizontal and straight and then bend the forearm lifting the orange. Repeat this with the other arm doing each exercise ten times.
3. Hand strength: get yourself a soft rubber ball or a squash ball. Squeeze the ball in each hand ten times.

These exercises should not be rushed and both the contraction and the relaxation are equally important so sitting down again after standing and letting the forearm down as well as contracting are equally important. Both the contraction and relaxation should take the same length of time. After a period of rest, up to five minutes, you can repeat this cycle of exercises again. As your strength and

▶

fitness improve you can increase your training up to about five cycles. Finish off each session with general flexibility exercises.

The principles of training to improve strength are that you gradually increase the resistance and number of repetitions. Only increase either the number of repetitions or the weight on any day; you should not increase the load by more than 10 per cent on any occasion. For the older person, we would be much more conservative in our advice and suggest that one should be very comfortable at each individual workload before increasing.

References

1 Fries JF. Physical activity, the compression of morbidity, and the health of the elderly. *J R Soc Med* 1996; **89**: 64–8.

2 Hagberg JM, Seals DR, Yerg JE. Metabolic responses to exercise in younger and older athletes and sedentary men. *J Appl Physiol* 1988; **65**: 900–908.

3 Tipton CM, Mathes RD, Maynard JA, Carey RA. The influence of physical activity on ligaments and tendons. *Med Sci Sports Exer* 1975; **7**: 165–75.

4 Young A, Stokes M, Crowe M. The size and strength of the quadriceps muscle of old and young men. *Clin Physiol* 1985; **5**: 145–54.

5 Pollock ML, Foster G, Knapp D *et al*. Effect of ageing and training on the aerobic capacity and body composition of master athletes. *J Appl Physiol* 1981; **1**: 87–9.

6 Vandervoort M, McComas AJ. Contractile changes in opposing muscles of the human ankle joint with ageing. *J Appl Physiol* 1986; **61**: 361–7.

7 MacAuley D, McCrum EE, Stott G *et al*. *The Northern Ireland Health and Activity Survey*. Government Publications, HMSO, 1994.

8 Fiatarone MA, O Neill EF, Ryan ND *et al*. Exercise training and nutritional supplementation for physical frailty in very elderly people. *N Engl J Med* 1994; **330**: 1769–75.

9 Fiatarone MA, Mars EC, Ryan ND *et al*. *JAMA* 1990; **263**: 3029–34.

10 ACSM American College of Sports Medicine Position Stand: The recommended quantity and quality of exercise for developing and maintaining cardiorespiratory and muscular fitness in healthy adults. *Med Sci Sports Exer* 1990; **22**: 265–74.

6 Children and exercise

Not only have overall population levels of physical activity declined, but there are signs of a serious decline in the level of physical activity among children and patterns established in early life are maintained as these children get older. More alarming than the decline in physical activity is evidence of declining levels of physical fitness and the relationship between poor physical activity, fitness and cardiovascular risk factors. Children are considerably less active than 10 or 20 years ago with correspondingly higher levels of obesity, lipids and hypertension.

The key component of cardiovascular health is aerobic fitness and British studies have shown poor levels of aerobic fitness in children of all ages. Physical activity in children is not helped either by changing patterns in education where children in Britain have the least curriculum time dedicated to physical education.

British children lead an inactive [1] life and it appears that they are becoming increasingly inactive. This pattern of inactivity has long-term health implications and even at school age there is evidence of the development of cardiovascular risk factors. From these findings one could postulate a relationship between childhood inactivity, adult inactivity and increased risk of ischaemic heart disease in later life. Activity levels in children drop considerably after the age of 14 years. In general boys are more active than girls at all ages and, after the age of 14 years, activity levels among girls drop very low. Activity levels are not homogenous and, at every age, there are some very active children but also a group who take virtually no exercise. One may guess as to the cause of this decline in physical activity. Certainly recent changes in education have changed the emphasis on physical education in school. Even though most physical activity (75%) was not at school, it remained a very important part of the overall exercise pattern and was the only exercise undertaken by 30% of pupils.

These findings are not confined to this country, however, and data from the United States 1990 Youth Risk Behavior Survey showed that most teenagers in grades 9 though 12 were not performing regular vigorous activity and about 50% were not enrolled in physical education activity classes. At age 12 years of age, 70% of children are active but by age 21 years, this falls to 42% of men and 30% of women. Findings are similar in the UK where children become far less active through adolescence, girls are less active than boys and become even less active than boys as they get older.

Simply encouraging children to be more active or highlighting the medical risks will be insufficient to change habits. There must be a coherent multidisciplinary strategy towards increasing physical activity. This must include schools and parents together with health care professionals. It should also apply more widely in facilitating young people to be more active by measures such as making it easier and safer to cycle to school, and reducing the sale of sports facilities by schools and local authorities. Town planning is important so that it is safe for children to cycle and play on the streets with access to leisure facilities close by. An increasing number of children are transported to school by car and bus and fewer walk or cycle. The active component of children's lives has been reduced and it is the ultimate irony that increasing numbers of people have to drive to leisure centres to exercise. Of course children's lifestyles are intricately woven in the lifestyle of their parents.

Obesity is increasing among children and this population obesity is essentially due to an imbalance between activity level and energy intake. Risk factor patterns track as people get older so that obese inactive children become obese inactive adults with all the associated risk factors. The increase in childhood obesity can be directly related to this increase in inactivity and this pattern of obesity tracks into later adult life such that there is an 80% likelihood of obese children becoming obese adults. There is little evidence to suggest that population obesity in this country is due to dietary fat, and indeed consumption of fat has decreased in recent years. Television is taking over from active sport and the big challenge will be in encouraging people to be more active. Activity levels are decreasing and the components of physical activity decrease in particular after the ages of 13–14 years old.

The research community has also focused its attention on children, showing that children are less fit now than they were in the past. They are more overweight and less active. The relationship between activity and cardiovascular risk factors is the same in children as it is in adults. Children who are fitter also have lower risk factors and more favourable lipid profiles. By increasing childhood level of activity we have a better chance of improving adult cardiovascular risk. It is essential, therefore, to establish favourable levels of activity in childhood. Information from studies which include comprehensive school-based health promotion and education intervention show improvements in risk factors.

There is a national policy towards promoting exercise and increasing physical activity among children. This is intended to reverse the increasing inactivity with its associated increase in cardiovascular and other risk factors. Children follow the role model of adults and the predominantly sedentary lifestyle of the adult population is reflected in children's inactivity. If there is an increase in physical activity among children there is also likely to be an increase in activity-related injury. Of course, most injuries are minor soft tissue injuries but it is difficult to establish the true incidence because of the difficulty in definition.

Risks of sport in children

At the other end of the activity spectrum are those talented children who participate in high level sport with intense training and competition schedules, and who may be subject to physical overuse injury and psychological stress. They are exposed to potential injury from overtraining or trauma. Sport is becoming more and more competitive and children are starting to train at younger and younger ages. There is concern about the risks such intense sport at a very young age and in particular the hazard of sport at a time when bones and joints may be most susceptible to injury. Between 3 and 22% of children are injured each year taking part in sport, with boys more often injured than girls [2]. There are difficulties in classifying injury which may partly explain the different injury rates between children and adults. Children may be injured differently and at different sites than adults.

One of the most important potential factors, however, is the difference between biological age and chronological age. With the changes in physical appearance and the growth spurt associated with puberty there is great variation in size between children of the same chronological age. Those children who had their growth spurt early and who are more physically advanced will be much bigger than their prepubertal contemporaries. Players selected according to chronological age will show great variation in size and it seems inappropriate to match these players together, especially in contact sports. It would be more appropriate to match them by biological or physiological criteria. Puberty is the time of most rapid bone growth and the site of injury in a young person may have serious long-term implications.

Injuries that cause the most problems are growth plate injuries. As general practitioners we are acutely aware of the implications of a growth plate injury on the long-term development of children. A growth plate injury leading to significant leg length discrepancy will give a child a limp, a physical impairment and a psychological burden for the remainder of their lives. In adolescent sport, the growth plate, joint surfaces and musculotendinous insertions are most at risk [3].

There may be other factors related to health that may leave children more liable to injury. The American Academy of Paediatrics [4] issued guidelines in 1988 on children's participation in sport as physicians were concerned about potential injury. The guidelines are addressed at those doctors performing preparticipation medical examinations. Because of the nature of various sports and the difficulty in issuing general guidelines which would be relevant and appropriate for all sports, they subdivided sports according to their exercise intensity, and the potential for collision.

Risks in elite sport

There was little objective evidence of the incidence and nature of injuries in children in the UK until the Training of Young Athletes (TOYA) study. This was a major prospective study of paediatric sports injuries. This study recruited 453 elite young athletes in five 2-year age groups from ages 8 to 16 years old and followed them for self reported sports injuries. The study was of four sports: tennis, gymnastics, swimming and soccer. The average incidence of sports injury per year was 54 per 100 athletes [5]. The lowest injury rate was found in swimmers (37%) and the greatest was in soccer players (67%). Most (70%) injuries were acute and minor. Only 4 of the 452 athletes reported that injury had been their reason for retiring from sport. The study concluded that most injuries in elite athletes were minor, the incidence was low and that injury did not, in the short or medium term, seem to be a significant health problem.

One may have expected a difference in injury related to intensity and frequency of training but there was, surprisingly, no related difference in the injury rates. They concluded that intensive training with good facilities and coaches is less likely to cause injury than unstructured sport in disorganised environment. This finding is in keeping with previously published work [6] comparing injuries in sport with free play. During this 2-year study there were 492 injuries reported of which one third were overuse type injuries and the remainder were due to trauma. General practitioners will find it interesting that most of these elite young athletes sought their sports injury health care outside the NHS.

The results of this study were in contrast to the expectations. In 1988 the same authors had expressed concern [7] about the possible harmful effects of exercise and intensive training in young people and about how juvenile athletes were already subjected to very high levels of training. They expected a large number of overuse injures but the findings of the study were rather different and they found that the most common injuries were due to trauma and the incidence was low. The concluded that sport in children was safe and that injuries were minor and self limiting. Over one half of the injuries were sustained outside the structured sport and such injuries were more likely to occur during some other activity. Rather than children being at more risk from intense highly active sport, highly organised sport seemed to be protective.

Balance of risks and benefits

How do we balance the risks and benefits of sport? The risks of participation in sport appear to be low. Children are often injured in play, so the relationship between sport and injury depends on the definition of sport. From the TOYA study, injury in children is relatively low and there are other risks far greater than that associated with high intensity exercise. With the increase in investment in facilities and medical support it is encouraging to note that those elite athletes who had access to quality facilities and good support sustained less serious injury but this is no reassurance to those who are less privileged. Put in comparison with the huge benefits of a healthy active lifestyle, the evidence clearly indicates that we should be encouraging children to be active. Clearly encouragement towards greater activity should be accompanied by investment in appropriate medical support.

Other factors

Children can also suffer psychological injury. Pressure for performance in children is usually primarily from their parents who may try to live vicariously through them, exerting immense pressure to succeed. The sacrifices that a child makes if they wish to succeed in top level sport are immense. They lose friends, albeit making some more during sport, but they spend long periods of time training when otherwise they might be reading or relaxing. Children also like to live up to adult expectations. They have adult role models as figures of authority and they will often tend to follow those instructions even when they are physiologically unable or the exercise is unsuitable for them.

The type of sport is also important. Children appear to have a different biochemical metabolism. They tend not to produce lactate. They may also be physiologically unsuitable for long periods of aerobic type activity. Shorter, more active, recreation may be more appropriate.

References

1 Riddoch C, Savage JM, Murphy N *et al*. Long term health implications of fitness and physical activity patterns. *Arch Dis Childh* 1991; **66**: 1426–33.
2 Helms PJ. Sports injuries in children: should we be concerned? *Arch Dis Child* 1997; **77**: 161–3.
3 Gerrard DF. Overuse injury and growing bones. The young athlete at risk. *Br J Sports Med* 198; **27**: 14–8.
4 Committee on sports medicine. Recommendations for participation in competitive sports. *Pediatrics* 1988; **81**: 737–9.
5 Baxter-Jones A, Maffuli N, Helms P. Low injury rates in elite athletes. *Arch Dis Childh* 1993; **68**: 130–2.
6 Micheli LJ, Klein JD. Sports injuries in children and adolescents. *Br J Sports Med* 1991; **25**: 6–9.
7 Maffuli N, Helms P. Controversies about intensive training in young athletes. *Arch Dis Childh* 1988; **63**: 1405–7.

7 Treating minor injuries

The general practitioner who wishes to become more involved in sport and agrees to become medical officer to a local club or team should make a particular effort to learn about the problems associated with the sport. As sports medicine evolves as a specialty it is becoming more important to seek further training in sport and exercise medicine. It is no longer enough simply to offer one's services as an interested spectator. Clubs and players expect their doctor to have further knowledge and expertise. Such expectations have medicolegal implications and already the medical defence organisations have noted an increase in inquiries with some leading to court appearances.

Treating minor injuries, sprains and strains

The general practitioner who offers his or her services as a sports doctor should be familiar with all phases of sports injury treatment, from managing the initial injury, right through to rehabilitation and prevention. You may be the doctor at the trackside or on the touchline and responsible for coordinating first aid. Indeed, in your role as medical officer you may be called upon to teach others the principles of first aid. Patients attending the surgery will, in most cases, have had first aid treatment before they attend, but it is important nevertheless to have a thorough understanding of management principles in case one is asked to act as team or event doctor. The basic principles of the treatment of minor sporting injuries are those that apply to any soft tissue injury. This chapter will deal with first aid management of soft tissue injuries in particular. The treatment plan, from the GP's perspective, will focus on second phase management and on rehabilitation in most cases.

Immediate treatment of soft tissue injuries

The aim of treatment is to reduce pain and swelling, and speed rehabilitation with the principal objective being a rapid return to sport. The mnemonic RICE indicates the key stages and the letters represent Rest, Ice, Compression and Elevation. These guidelines apply to minor injuries only, and if there is any doubt about diagnosis the athlete should, of course, be investigated further.

Rest!

Rest is relative and rehabilitation is early. An injury needs rest but this is rest of that injured part and does not mean total inactivity. For example a leg injury, such as a sprained ankle, may prevent running but should not prevent swimming, upper body circuits or weight training. Maintaining cardiovascular fitness is important so that the athlete can return to the same level or performance or as close to that level as is possible after injury. While cardiovascular fitness is transferable and can be maintained by cross training, the athlete will be keen to return to sport-specific exercise. This too is possible without weight bearing. For example a runner can run in the pool wearing a flotation jacket and mimic closely the specific muscle movement of running without impact or the fear of re-injury.

Ice

Ice cools the skin and underlying tissue. This reduces swelling, helps prevent bruising, and has some pain relieving effect. Ice can be applied in whatever form: ice cubes in a bag, bags of frozen peas, proprietary iced strapping and pads, or simple ice application. The ice should be wrapped in a damp towel to avoid direct contact between the ice and skin. If not, the direct application of ice may burn the skin. Ice application should be repeated every 2–3 minutes for about 20 minutes. Those who act as team doctors or who are responsible for providing medical advice to a sports club or organisation should ensure that ice is always available at both the training ground and competition site. Common sense suggests that the ice should not be kept in the fridge in the bar, which will have restricted opening times. If ice is not available, cold clean fresh running water may be a substitute. It is the cooling effect that is most important.

Compression

Swelling begins almost immediately after injury. This may be due to bleeding at first but it also occurs in the absence of bleeding when it is due to oedema and local tissue inflammation. This swelling can be reduced by pressure, usually in the form of a bandage or pressure dressing. After initial treatment with ice the injured limb should be strapped for compression. It is important, of course, to ensure that this compression is not so tight that it inhibits blood supply. An elasticated support bandage such as Tubigrip may be sufficient but a crepe bandage is inadequate as it loosens very quickly.

Elevation

Fluid runs downhill. Raising the injured limb, ideally above waist height, minimises swelling. By raising the limb we reduce both the accumulation of fluid in a dependent limb and aid venous return.

This first stage of management occurs at the track side or in the changing room but the success of this initial management also depends greatly on the injured athlete and how they react in the first 24 hours. The aim of the first phase of treatment is to relieve pain and reduce swelling. After first aid it is very important that the injured athlete does not undo all the good initial treatment by heading off to the bar and standing for hours imbibing further anaesthetic! After standing for a few hours that sprained ankle will become more swollen, immobile and recovery and rehabilitation will be greatly delayed.

Analgesia and anti-inflammatory medication

In most cases simple analgesia using paracetamol is effective in reducing pain. Non-steroidal anti-inflammatory (NSAID) medication may be used as an adjunct in short-term pain relief, but is often used in long-term management. NSAIDs do have side effects, however, with possible gastroduodenal bleeding or perforation. The NSAIDs least likely to cause problems are ibuprofen, naproxen and diclofenac [1] and both ibuprofen and diclofenac have short half lives so they may be more suitable for intermittent pain. For those at risk of gastroduodenal problems, H_2 antagonists such as ranitidine may be useful.

Misoprostol may protect against upper gastrointestinal problems and reduce ulceration (200 μg q.d.s.).

Pattern of injury

When a player is injured, even with a minor muscle injury or ankle sprain, there will inevitably be some impairment of function. This may be a direct result of injury to the muscle or through impairment of the proprioceptive response after an injury to the joint capsule. When this occurs there is an increased likelihood of further injury, as the mechanism of reaction to physical stress will be impaired. The player may be keen to play on and the injury relatively minor but the likelihood of a second, possibly much more serious, injury remains. The likelihood of an injury occurring following a previous injury is known as the second injury syndrome.

Injuries are more likely to occur in team games when the players are tired. Hence we see the pattern of increased injury in the latter stages of the second half of a match. By this time the players are tired, mentally and physically. With tired muscles the response to proprioceptive stimuli may be subtly impaired, the body may not react as quickly and injury can occur. It is difficult to apply a medical answer to this problem other than to encourage a preventative strategy of improved fitness to allow players to cope with the stresses of the later stages of the game.

Muscle soreness

Muscle soreness is almost an inevitable part of exercise and training. Those who increase their training load or intensity often suffer some delayed onset muscle soreness (DOMS). This is not a severe acute injury with localised tenderness but is a generalised ache in those muscles used in the exercise. This usually reflects microscopic muscle damage; the pain and stiffness is due to release of muscle enzymes from damaged muscle cells. Muscle enzyme release may be reflected in an elevation of creatine kinase. Muscle soreness may be minimised by moderate planned increase in exercise load. A warm-down period can help wash out the breakdown products of muscle damage and return to gentle activity can help restore muscle function.

Contusions

A direct blow on a muscle may cause bruising and bleeding within muscle tissue. Blood leaks around the muscle tissue and causes pain and swelling within the muscle belly. This may lead to a partial or complete paralysis so the muscle is less effective. With a major contusion there is severe pain, the muscle will not contract, and the player cannot continue to play. Less severe injuries will disable a player who, although they can continue to play, is less effective and more likely to sustain a second injury. Typically a contusion injury occurs in the thigh where athletes may call it a 'Charley horse' or 'dead leg'. On examination the muscle feels tense and tender and the athlete cannot extend it over its full range of movement. The priority in early treatment is to reduce the swelling and bleeding within the muscle and, as with any muscle injury, first principles apply. There should be no further vigorous muscle activity or forced passive stretching as this may restart bleeding and extend the damage. Non-steroidal anti-inflammatory medication can help reduce pain and bleeding.

With such a contusion injury there is often a delay in return to sport and the risk of myositis ossificans. Reduction of the pain and swelling and return to full range of movement may take 2–3 weeks, even with the most effective treatment. If the swelling does not reduce and the range of muscle remains limited then one must exclude myositis ossificans. Myositis ossificans is the calcification of the organised haematoma with formation of new bone within the muscle tissue. This has serious implications for the athlete who cannot return to training or competition. On clinical examination the muscle swelling may not have completely resolved and there is palpable swelling within the muscle. This forms a sausage shaped hard swelling deep within the muscle belly. Calcification is first seen on X-ray about 2–3 weeks after the injury. If the swelling remains, if an injury fails to heal or there is any sign of calcification on the X-ray, the patient should see a specialist orthopaedic surgeon. Treatment is usually by surgical removal of the calcified mass, followed by an extended period of rehabilitation. This is a relatively unusual injury but when it occurs it causes major morbidity and delay in rehabilitation.

Physiotherapy

The process of recovery from injury begins with first aid. After initial management the main focus is on functional rehabilitation. Many injuries damage muscle and inhibit muscle function. Physiotherapy offers various treatments which may speed muscle recovery at local cellular and gross muscle level. These include ultrasound, various electrical treatments and lasers. Perhaps the most important tool of the physiotherapist, however, is the hands-on practical approach. In most cases the physiotherapist is the key person for coordinating treatment and advice on rehabilitation and suitable retraining. Their training gives them particular understanding of the structure and function of muscle, optimum retraining and specific exercises in recovery but, while they may have sophisticated equipment available the most important attribute will be their knowledge and understanding of the needs of the sport. In the management of acute soft tissue injury in practice, the physiotherapist is the most useful local community resource.

Warm-up

Warm-up, as the name suggests, is a gradual and progressive exercise programme at the beginning of training or before competition which increases blood flow to the muscle and increases muscle temperature. All athletes, whatever the sport, should undertake a progressive warm-up routine, beginning with some gentle activity to increase muscle blood flow and increasing in intensity to submaximal level before full activity. In a cold environment it is also important to wear sufficient appropriate clothing to increase and then maintain body temperature, and especially local muscle temperature. Special clothing is available, designed for sport, which can retain heat and is especially useful for those training and racing in cool temperatures. The purpose of a warm-up is to raise muscle temperature which improves biochemical efficiency, elasticity and muscle plasticity.

Stretching

Stretching should be an integral part of the strategy for prevention of and rehabilitation from injury. There are different objectives in prevention and rehabilitation. In prevention, we aim to extend the range of muscle movement so that a muscle will not be torn by sudden contraction at the limit of its range This is especially important in sprinting or where there are sudden changes in speed or direction of play, as in field games.

Stretching as part of rehabilitation has a different function. After muscle injury there is bleeding which organises. There is invasion of fibroblasts and deposition of collagen. The muscle heals but with deposition of scar tissue. After injury the muscle is usually shortened and the scar tissue lacks the plasticity of normal muscle. Stretching during the recovery phase helps align fibres in the direction of movement and allows the tissue to lengthen. It allows recovery to the original length and range of movement and thus helps reduce the likelihood of further injury.

Static stretching is the gradual lengthening of a muscle by slowly extending the muscle over the range of movement. It is specific and stretches the muscle only in the actual direction of stretching. A more effective form of stretching which uses the normal physiological muscle response after contraction is Proprioceptive Neuromuscular Facilitation (PNF). Using this technique one contracts the muscle and then uses the compensatory relaxation phase immediately after contraction in order to stretch. Each contraction should be held for about 10 seconds and then the muscle extended and stretched immediately afterwards for about 10 seconds. Stretching should be included as an integral part of every training session as the benefits of stretching only persist if it is continued. Cold muscles are less pliable so muscles should not be stretched when cold. This is especially important in cold weather. Stretching is best performed after a short period of general light activity to warm-up, when the muscle blood flow has been increased and the temperature of the muscle has been raised slightly. We still see trainers encouraging and athletes performing ballistic stretching. This stimulates the stretch reflex which causes an involuntary contraction and one cannot stretch a contracted muscle.

A muscle is most effective in the middle of its range of movement. Stretching aims to increase this effective middle range of movement. It also helps to lengthen the muscle so that sudden contractions at the limit of the range are less likely to tear the muscle. A warm muscle is more pliable and supple so the athlete should warm the muscle tissue before stretching. This is particularly important in cold weather, when a muscle is cold and stiff. The most effective method of warming muscle tissue is to increase blood flow in the capillaries by light exercise during a warm-up. The purpose of a warm-up is not to achieve a training effect but is simply to increase circulation to the large muscle groups. The intensity is therefore unimportant, and should be sufficient only to increase blood flow. In cold environmental conditions it is important to maintain muscle temperature afterwards so heat should be retained by wearing appropriate clothing such as a tracksuit or thermal clothing. Recently, close fitting long shorts and tights have become popular and these may indeed have some heat retaining properties. After a gentle warm-up which need last no longer than 5–10 minutes depending on the environmental conditions, the athlete can begin a stretching routine. This should include all the main muscle groups to be used in the sport and should be unhurried.

Each muscle should be extended slowly and progressively and there is no place for painful passive stretching or bouncing. In the past, athletes have been seen doing rapid short stretching. This has no effect other than to stimulate the stretch reflex with the associated muscle contraction which defeats the purpose of stretching. The major muscle groups to stretch in the legs are the hamstrings, quadriceps group, adductors and calf.

Calf stretches

Lean against a wall or fixed surface with one leg extended and the knee straight and the other leg forward and the knee bent. This allows one to stretch both the soleus and gastrocnemius. Relax the arms and feel the stretching at the calf. With the muscle extended, stretch and hold for 10 seconds, then relax (Figure 7.1).

A more effective method of stretching is to make use of the natural relaxation phase that occurs after every muscle contraction. This is called PNF or proprioceptive neuromuscular facilitation. Gently move to a position of slight tension on the calf muscle. Contract the muscle and hold for 10 seconds, then stretch the muscle and hold for 10 seconds, then relax. This sequence can be performed with all stretching exercises.

Hamstring stretches

The hamstrings can be stretched either sitting or standing (Figure 7.2). Sit on the floor with one leg extended and the other tucked underneath. Stretch out the corresponding arm and feel the stretch of the hamstring. Using PNF, one should first contract

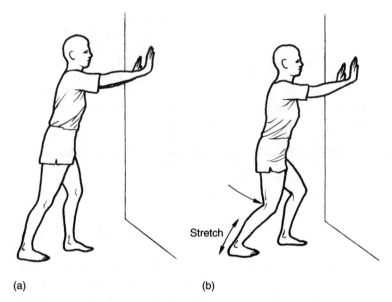

(a)   (b)

Figure 7.1 Calf stretching: (a) starting position and (b) stretching the calf.

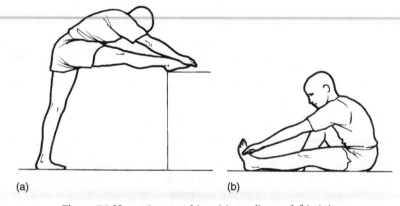

(a)   (b)

Figure 7.2 Hamstring stretching: (a) standing and (b) sitting.

the muscle against the floor, hold for 10 seconds and then stretch. The hamstring muscle group may also be stretched by putting the foot on a raised object: chair, hurdle or bar. Similarly the muscle can be stretched using the same PNF sequence.

Quadriceps stretches

Standing on one leg the foot is held behind the body and drawn upwards. One should feel some tension in the quadriceps muscle at the front of the thigh (Figure 7.3).

Adductor stretches

The adductors can also be stretched standing or using a raised bar, object or low hurdle (Figure 7.4).

Back stretches

The back and abdominal muscles can be stretched together. Flexibility of the lower spine is essential in prevention of many sports injuries where the back is loaded, from rowing to the rugby scrum. While standing, rotate the trunk from side to side and increase the range of movement of the arc.

A more specific exercise for flexion and extension can be undertaken using the floor. Take the position as if doing a press-up. Arch the back forming a high bridge. Hold for 10 seconds and then return to the normal position. Reverse the movement by bending back the shoulders neck and back so that the stomach is close to the floor. Similarly hold for 10 seconds and relax (Figure 7.5).

Shoulder stretches

The rotator cuff moves the shoulder in many directions. First one can generally mobilise the shoulder by shrugging the shoulders and rotating the shoulders slowly drawing circles with the arms. A more specific exercises for stretching at the end of the range of movement is by stretching the arm up the back and down the back as far as possible. This can be done using both arms together. Place one arm behind the back reaching upwards and the other arm over the top of the shoulder to meet it. Hold for 10 seconds and relax. Repeat for the other side (Figure 7.6).

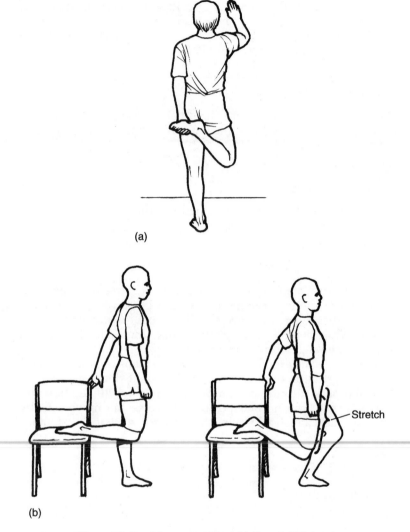

Figure 7.3 Quadriceps stretching: (a) fit and (b) injured.

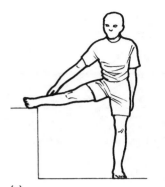
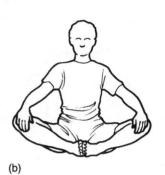

(a)   (b)

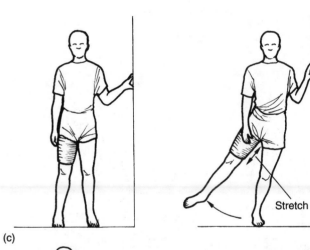

Stretch

(c)

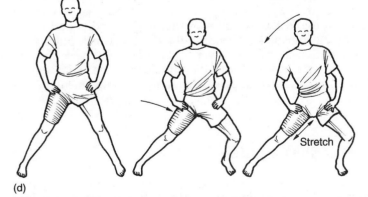

Stretch

(d)

Figure 7.4 Adductor stretching: (a) standing; (b) sitting; (c) gentle adductor stretch for rehabilitation after injury and (d) next stage of rehabilitation.

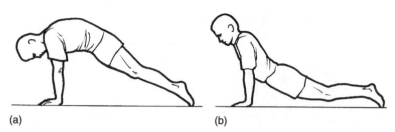

(a)   (b)

Figure 7.5 Back stretching: (a) arching the back and (b) contracting.

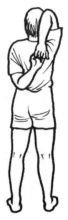

Figure 7.6 Shoulder stretching.

Neck stretches

Neck mobility and flexibility are important in some sports. Rotate the neck by drawing circles with your head. Increase the arc but avoid the extremes of the range. Flexion and extension may be stretched by bending the neck forward, putting the chin on the chest and backwards. Laterally the neck may be flexed with the ear towards the shoulders. The older person should avoid the extremes of the range of movement in this exercise.

Covert serious injuries

Even with a seemingly trivial injury, a more serious injury may lurk undetected. A sprain may be a fracture, concussion may lead to subdural haemorrhage, or a knee injury may be a ruptured cruciate. The immediate care of even the most apparently trivial injury demands conscientious and careful management.

The athletic injury history checklist

There is often a pattern of injury readily identifiable with a particular sport. To provide a comprehensive template for history and examination that would cover every eventuality in every sport would be impossible. The checklist below is simply an *aide-*

Athletic history checklist

Name:

Age:

Sport:

History of the injury:

Onset, exacerbating and relieving factors, relationship to the sport:

Previous consultations with other physicians, chiropracters, physiotherapists. (Athletes will often see various qualified and non-qualified specialists and may equate diagnosis and management independent of background):

Previous investigations:

Previous treatments:

Sporting history:

Type of sport, level of achievement, training history. Position on pitch, particular features of this position:

Changes in training – increase, decrease, changes in types of exercises. (It is helpful to have some understanding of the sport and the type of training that is entailed.):

Equipment – alteration in equipment such as change in position of bike, type of oars or position in boat, type or change in racquet, change in shoes, boots:

Examination – site-specific examination:

---

memoire, a reminder of the major important features of an athletic history. Those doctors who are involved with medical care in sport will modify this checklist to suit their own needs.

Reference

1 Rational use of NSAIDs for musculoskeletal disorders. *Drug Therap Bull* 1994; **32**: 91–5.

8 Emergencies

Sport is for fun but emergencies in sport can be life threatening. Dealing with such emergencies may not be sports medicine in the traditional sense, but all those involved with sport should be able to cope with any life threatening event. The importance of emergency care is also reflected in the increasing significance placed on the management of sports emergencies both in teaching courses and sports medicine examinations. In the scenario tests of the Diploma in Sports Medicine of the Scottish Royal Colleges for example, candidates are required to deal with simulated emergencies taking place where there are other environmental, metabolic or traumatic factors: the diabetic rambler who is injured in a fall on a remote highland glen, or the drug abusing cyclist who crashes during a long summer stage race. Emergencies do not occur in straightforward circumstances; sporting patients do not generally collapse in a hospital environment where there is convenient immediate access to the cardiac crash team The principles of emergency medicine are the same but many factors influence care in the sporting environment.

Emergency care

Learning how to deal with cardiac emergencies from a book is probably the least effective way to learn. Practical hands-on experience and tutoring by recognised experts is much more effective. This section is written, therefore, as an *aide-memoire* and is no substitute for tuition. There are increasing numbers of ATLS and BASICs courses for prehospital care. If you unable to attend such courses, you may like to contact your local ambulance training unit where the instructor can put you through your paces. As part of emergency care it is essential to become familiar not just with cardiac resuscitation but with other aspects of management of emergencies.

Cardiopulmonary resuscitation

Cardiopulmonary resuscitation (CPR) is based on the same principles irrespective of the situation or environment. Coronary artery disease is the major cause of death in the developed word, many of which deaths are sudden and unpredictable. Clearly sporting patients are not in the high-risk group, from an epidemiological perspective, but this type of emergency does occur.

In sudden cardiac death the initial problem is usually a rhythm disorder, progressing to ventricular fibrillation and asystole. The two best predictors of survival are the nature of the rhythm disorder and time to defibrillation. This is the logic behind provision of portable defibrillators. Immediate defibrillation is unlikely in the sporting context, and maintaining circulation through CPR is often the only available option. The public are increasingly interested in learning CPR with pressure on doctors to teach CPR to many community groups. There is merit in learning CPR as good CPR improves survival and the public should be encouraged to learn the correct method.

Cardiopulmonary resuscitation is a combination of artificial ventilation and assisted circulation though external chest compression. Contrary to public perception, and although the actual mechanics are probably irrelevant, this assisted circulation is due to the changes in cardiothoracic pressure during the upstroke rather than the actual compression on the ventricle.

It is impossible to deal with CPR adequately in this book so readers are advised to consult a specialist text and to keep themselves up to date by attending regular training and retraining programmes.

Sudden cardiac death in sport

Sudden death in sport always makes news headlines. Because it most often occurs in the young athletic population, where death from any cause is least expected, and because it may occur in a very public environment, it attracts considerable media interest. This is in contrast to everyday deaths from other causes. As a result, general practitioners will be asked about the risks of sport or may be asked to comment publicly for the media.

The first historical reference to sudden death is probably that of Pheidippides who died after running the first 'marathon' from Athens to Marathon in 490 BC, bringing news of the of the victory over the Persians. During the late 1970s and 1980s there was a huge running boom, and the parallel belief that running provided the complete antidote to ischaemic heart disease. Indeed, a celebrated paper by Bassler [1] suggested that marathon running provided complete protection against heart disease and that fatal coronary artery disease had never been found in a marathon runner. This hypothesis was later proved incorrect [2]. Exercise does reduce the overall statistical risk of ischaemic heart disease, and those who undertake endurance type training are less likely to develop coronary artery disease, but there is none-the-less a slightly increased risk of sudden death while actually participating in sport.

Prevention of sudden cardiac death

Patients are encouraged to have a medical examination before participating in sport, especially those over 40 years of age. It is, however, difficult to predict those at risk as sudden death occurs often in those with asymptomatic heart disease. Physical examination and ECG screening may detect some high risk individuals but screening is unlikely to detect disease in those who are asymptomatic. False positives can occur with resting ECGs and a normal resting and exercise ECG does not always exclude cardiovascular disease. For any screening programme the sensitivity, specificity and prevalence must be related to the outcome and it is difficult to justify pre-exercise cardiac screening under these mathematical constraints.

For the older sports participant we would recommend sport appropriate to age and general level of fitness. Sport should be regular, submaximal and rhythmical and the intensity progression should be gradual. All older participants should avoid sudden high intensity and isometric exercise such as squash or weightlifting. Symptoms such as chest pain or extreme fatigue should not be ignored. Smoking should be avoided because of its more immediate effect on free fatty acids, catecholamine release and its arrythmogenic effects especially in the postexercise period. A warm-down is essential as the postexercise period is of particular high risk for arrythmia. Athletes with heart conditions can be found competing at a very high level, even with a serious cardiac condition, as they may be asymptomatic. The value of the preparticipation medical examination is unknown.

Northcote [3] believed that 80% of sudden deaths could be avoided by posing six questions which would select high risk individuals who should have a detailed medical examination. He pointed out that it is the macho response to middle age which leads men to dangerous and violent sports. These questions will select those who should have further investigation.

Pre-exercise screening questions

- Age over 60?
- Self or a relative have diabetes?
- Smoke?
- Hypertensive?
- Symptoms of chest pain, tightness, discomfort, breathlessness or palpitations?
- Family history of ischaemic heart disease?

Viral illness

Athletes should not train or compete when suffering from a significant viral illness. A viraemia may be associated with a myocarditis and exercise may precipitate an arrythmia. Coxsackie B has been implicated in animal studies of myocarditis and it is suggested that 25% of patients with true influenza also have some degree of myocarditis. It is reasonable to suspect that those suffering from a viral illness who have muscular aches and pains may also have some myocardial inflammation. Those who have a temperature, or whose illness is accompanied by muscular aches and pains, should not exercise.

Other factors may drive an athlete to compete. In the major mass participation events peer pressure or pressure of sponsorship may influence some to participate when unwell.

Cardiac hazards of exercise

One of the major reasons for promoting exercise is the evidence of a reduction in death from cardiovascular disease associated with physical activity seen in large epidemiological studies. It is difficult, therefore, to reconcile these cardiovascular benefits with the deaths that occur during exercise. While exercise can indeed protect against cardiovascular disease, there is the paradox of an increased likelihood of sudden death while actually participating in this activity. Sudden cardiac death associated with sport is a tragic event and is a particularly difficult concept to explain in the context of general practice where our relationship is with an individual patient and not with improving population statistics.

Injury can also occur as a result of sports participation and has a major cost both to the individual and the state [4]. The benefits of exercise must always be balanced against the costs in financial, emotional and physical terms. The slogan that 'sport for all' means 'sports injury for all' remains.

Estimating the risk of sudden cardiac death in sport

When we encourage patients to exercise, they often ask us about the risks and hazards and can quote anecdotes or news stories about such events. There is a risk, difficult to quantify, although certainly small in relation to the undoubted benefits, but a risk nevertheless. Among young athletes, these events are rare with an estimated 0.75 and 0.13 deaths per 100,000 men and women per year, which is a risk of 1 per 133,000 men and 1 per 769,000 women [5]. For exercise-related cardiac death in healthy adults at any age in the United States the incidence is still low at 5.4 deaths per 100,000 or a rate of 1 death for every 18,000 men [6]. Other work suggests an incidence of 1 death per 15,000 previously healthy joggers [7] and in this study the relative risk of sudden death in joggers was seven times higher for joggers than in other activities.

As these events occur infrequently, it is often difficult to collect high quality data but we have evidence from a number of studies which help us identify the most common causes. About one in 10 sudden deaths in young people are associated with sport, but it is a relatively rare event overall and estimates from the United States suggest that it occurs in 1 in 200,000 athletes. Exercise-related death in the young appears to have a different pattern and aetiology from that in middle age. In young people, exercise-related death is usually not associated with degenerative atherosclerotic disease and such deaths are unlikely to have been as a direct result of the sport or activity. Exercise may, however, trigger death due to an underlying condition.

Data from the United States suggest that the most common cause of death is hypertrophic cardiomyopathy (HOCM), although death can occur due other congenital conditions such as coronary arteries abnormalities. Conduction defects are cited as a common cause but post-mortem diagnosis of such conditions is very difficult.

It is very difficult to collect information on sudden death in sport in order to estimate the magnitude of the problem. In one of the most important studies from the USA the author [8] gathered together information, on those who had died suddenly, from a number of sources including registers, news accounts and other information sources. He found that of 158 deaths, 24 (15%) were attributable to non-cardiovascular causes leaving 134. Of the 120 men, death may have been due to a heterogenous spectrum of cardiovascular disease, most commonly HOCM. He also believed that the preparticipation medical examination would be of limited value in identification of underlying cardiovascular abnormalities.

In another of the better quality studies from the United States, the causes of death in a study of 100 cardiac deaths in young people [5], were as follows; hypertrophic cardiomyopathy in 58%, coronary artery anomalies in 13%, myocarditis in 7%, aortic stenosis in 6% and dilated cardiomyopathy in 6%. Recognition of HOCM as the major cause of sudden death has lead to calls for screening. The condition occurs in 2 per 1000 adults aged 25–35 years old, and screening for the condition would not fulfil the appropriate criteria for a national screening programme. There is little evidence that it would be effective in detecting HOCM and preventing death. Selective screening of relatives of those with HOCM using echocardiography would, however, be appropriate as it is a congenital condition (being autosomal dominant).

Marfans syndrome, a connective tissue disorder, is another genetic condition which has been implicated in sudden cardiac death. The diagnosis should be much easier because of the physical manifestations of the condition. Height is the main physical sign, but there are other associated connective tissue abnormalities and weaknesses which may give rise to a ruptured aortic aneurysm and mitral valve disease. Athletes with this condition are likely to self select into sports where height is a particular advantage such as basketball, volleyball and high jumping and there have been celebrated deaths of major stars from cardiac problems related to Marfans. The condition is rare in the general population, but has an increased frequency in such sports where those at risk should be screened by echocardiography and may be excluded from sport. Routine echocardiography is a feature of medical examinations in some of these sports such as professional basketball.

Of conduction defects, Wolff–Parkinson–White syndrome is a potential cause of death as the accessory conduction pathway bypassing the Bundle of His may give rise to ventricular rhythm abnormalities. It has a prevalence of 1:1000 so is likely to be prevalent in the sporting population. If the condition is detected, the patients should be assessed by a cardiologist with a view to possible treatment and may be advised to have radioablation. Myocarditis is another condition often cited as a possible cause of sudden death but, once again, post-mortem diagnosis is extremely difficult.

Many athletes, and indeed physicians, are confused in trying to differentiate between the physiological hypertrophy that occurs in endurance sports and the hypertrophy that occurs in HOCM. It is important to emphasise that the training effect of endurance exercise on the ventricular wall is quite different from that which occurs in HOCM. Exercise-related hypertrophy occurs in the left ventricle whereas septal hypertrophy is the classic finding in HOCM. The diagnostic challenge is in the asymptomatic athlete where making the correct diagnosis may have dramatic implications. Physiological hypertrophy is simply a training effect and the athlete can continue training but the athlete with HOCM risks death. For the general practitioner the family history and clinical findings are critical. Those with a family history should always be screened, but others may be detected in routine or pretraining medical examinations. Any athlete with a cardiac murmur should be investigated, and in view of the difficulties in diagnosis, a specialist cardiology opinion should be sought. Electrocardiographic changes are difficult to differentiate but echocardiographic findings of septal thickness exceeding 15 mm and a small left ventricular cavity are considered diagnositic.

Pre-exercise screening

Medical screening does not hold all the answers [9]. It is difficult to detect HOCM on clinical examination. The only pointer to diagnosis is a systolic murmur that is accentuated by the Valsalva manoeuvre or on squatting. One cannot detect anomalous coronary artery lesions on examination but it should be kept in mind in the differential diagnosis of any athlete with chest pain on exertion. While there is no evidence to indicate that echocardiography is valuable as a screening tool it is relatively simple and inexpensive and may become more commonplace in the future [10,11]. One could also argue that, in the context of sudden athletic death, a defibrillator should be standard equipment for the team doctor and athletic trainer.

A recent study [12] of prospective screening of 5,615 high school athletes in the United States illustrates some of the problems associated with screening. In this study they found 22 athletes who qualified for exclusion from sport or who required further evaluation. Using criteria for identifying 'at risk' individuals agreed at the Bethesda conference [13], they detected no patients on history alone, 1 in 6,000 on examination, 1 in 1000 on blood pressure and 1 in 350 on electrocardiograph (ECG). They concluded that the ECG was by far the most effective screening tool. Of course, the prevalence of cardiac abnormalities is very low and the authors of this study suggest that the prevalence of HOCM in high school athletes would be 50 in a total of 2.1 million or 1 in 40,000 and the overall prevalence of cardiovascular abnormalities with potential to cause sudden death would be 1 in 20,000. That the prevalence in the athletic population was less than the general population (1 in 500) suggests some self selection or preselection. It would be very expensive to screen such a large population and it is likely that the cost would be greatly increased if one were to include the cost of investigating false positives. The subject of screening always creates controversy. The authors of this paper recognise the difficulties but recommend that if the objective is to reduce the number of non-traumatic sudden deaths each high school athlete should have an ECG at least once.

The risks of exercise in adults

A recent review [14], indicates that the absolute incidence of exercise death is 0.75 and 0.13 per 100,000 of young men and women athletes and 6 per 100,000 of middle-aged men during exertion each year. From 4% to 20% of acute myocardial infarctions were associated with moderate or heavy physical exertion which suggests that the annual rate of exercise-related myocardial infarction could range from 1 per 571 to 3,714 men per year.

The pattern of sports-related death in adults is different from sudden cardiac death in young people. As with all adults, the most common cause of sudden death during exercise [15] is coronary artery disease but other causes include cardiomyopathies, cerebrovascular events and aortic dissection. A recent review [16] suggested that acute myocardial infarction may occur in exercise as a result of atherosclerotic plaque rupture, a paradoxical acute vasoconstriction with exercise, or through platelet activation with a reduced fibrinolytic response and reduced prostacyclin release [17,18]. The final event, in those with known coronary heart disease, is most likely to be ventricular fibrillation.

Exercise may a trigger a myocardial infarction and in one major study, the Multicentre Investigation of Limitation of Infarct Size study (MILIS), physical activity was implicated as a major risk factor since 14% reported moderate physical activity and 9% reported vigorous activity prior to infarct [19]. There are limitations to the conclusions that can be drawn from an observational study and the Myocardial Infarction Onset Study (MIOS) used a control group to try to establish relative risk. While 4.4% of those suffering a myocardial infarction reported heavy exertion within an hour of their infarction [20], they concluded that it was unaccustomed heavy exertion that was the precipitating cause. For those that were habitually active the risk was greatly reduced and there was an inverse relationship so that the relative risk of acute myocardial infarction was 2.4 (95% CI 1.5–3.7) in those who were active on five or more occasions per week, but was considerably greater in those who were inactive at 107 (95% CI 65–171).

It is important to emphasise that the absolute risk is low. The risk in cardiac patients is 1:60,000 but the risk in the general population is 1:565,000 person hours of vigorous activity [21]. Based on the current evidence, we can make some suggestions to those undertaking an exercise programme, and to those who give advice on exercise. Participants should be advised about the relative risk, their individual risk, and the benefits of exercise. They should be advised about the type, intensity and pattern of exercise that would be most suitable. Those in a high risk group should be advised about the importance of an appropriate warm-up, that exercise should be of moderate intensity, that they should also perform an appropriate warm-down and that they must stop if they have symptoms. Those unaccustomed to exercise and with known cardiac disease should avoid sudden vigorous unaccustomed exercise. The risk of myocardial infarction is always greatest in the morning but evidence from post-coronary rehabilitation programmes suggests that there is no evidence to confirm a greater risk for those who exercise in the morning in comparison to those attending in the afternoon [22].

Since most sudden cardiac deaths in adults are related to coronary artery disease, it would seem reasonable to explore the possibility of screening asymptomatic adults prior to undertaking an exercise programme. The American College of Sports Medicine recommends selective screening of those at high risk and in this group they include men over 40 years of age, women over 50 years of age, and individuals with more than one coronary risk factor. In addition, those with known coronary heart disease should undergo exercise testing before undertaking a vigorous exercise programme. A review [14] of studies of screening programmes suggest that they are expensive and ineffective. The exercise stress test is insufficiently sensitive to detect those at risk, and has an unacceptably high false positive rate. Surprisingly, a high risk strategy is also limited.

Cardiac rehabilitation

There is a general belief that moderate exercise can improve the long-term outlook in symptomatic ischaemic heart disease and evidence that exercise improves the physiological parameters. Cardiac rehabilitation programmes after myocardial infarction are of particular importance. Modest activity, such as daily walking, is of low risk. Some programmes aim for a more ambitious level of activity, even up to completing a marathon, but low intensity exercise may be as effective as higher intensity aerobic activity even up to one year [23]. Specific exercise guidelines have been published by the American College of Cardiology [24]. The protective effect of exercise only lasts while the individual continues the exercise programme.

The athlete's heart

There is still some confusion among the public, and indeed the medical profession, about the athlete's heart and the difficulties of differentiating between physiolgical and pathological cardiac enlargement. The athlete's heart was first described by Henschen [25] almost 100 years ago and has perplexed cardiologists ever since. It is a physiological adaptation, but the features so mimic pathological hypertrophic cardiomyopathy that doubts often arise. A recent review [26] highlighted some of the problems. The physiological adaptation associated with endurance type training includes left ventricular hypertrophy and an increase in end diastolic volume. These changes are most marked in high intensity endurance sports such as cycling. In contrast, the changes seen on echocardiography associated with hypertrophic cardiomyopathy include asymmetric hypertrophy, abnormal filling and small cavity size. There is, however, some overlap in the features of both conditions which lead cardiologists to explore more definitive methods of identifying the pathological and it is likely that further refinements to magnetic resonance techniques will aid diagnosis.

Guidelines on medical examination

It is difficult for the general practitioner to know how to proceed when asked to advise on the preparticipation medical examination. There are no useful British guidelines but a panel of experts at the American Heart Association reviewed [27,28] the problems associated with screening young athletes and produced consensus recommendations based on the evidence. Their aim was 'to provide medical clearance for participation in competitive sports through routine and systematic evaluations intended to identify clinically relevant and pre-existing cardiovascular abnormalities and thereby reduce the risks associated with organised sports'. What should be done when abnormalities are detected was previously agreed at the Bethesda conference [29]. The conclusions of this paper appear to be in conflict with the evidence presented within the paper. They presented little evidence to show that screening would be effective, but recommended screening nevertheless.

For young athletes they recommended a complete personal and family history and physical examination. The examination was to identify or raise suspicion of those cardiovascular lesions known to cause sudden death or disease progression in young athletes. They recommended a history and physical examination before participation in sport at high school or college and that this should be repeated every two years. In the interim year a history should be obtained. The history should include questions to detect the following [27].

- Prior occurrence of exercise-related chest pain/discomfort or syncope/ near syncope as well as excessive, unexpected or unexplained shortness of breath or fatigue associated with exercise.
- Past detection of a heart murmur or increased blood pressure.
- Family history of premature death (sudden or otherwise), or significant disability from cardiovascular disease in a close relative younger than 50 years old or specific knowledge of the occurrence of certain conditions (e.g. hypertrophic cardiomyopathy, dilated cardiomyopathy, long QT interval. Marfan syndrome or clinically important arrythmias).

The physical examination should emphasise (but not necessarily be limited to) the following.

- Precordial ausculation in both the supine and standing positions to identify, in particular, heart murmurs consistent with dynamic left ventricular outflow obstruction.
- Assessment of the femoral artery pulses to exclude coarctation of the aorta.
- Recognition of the physical signs of Marfans Syndrome.
- Blood pressure.

It is also recommended that exercise stress tests should be performed selectively in men over 40 and women over 50 years of age.

References

1 Bassler TJ. Marathon running and immunity to atherosclerosis. *Ann N Y Acad Sci* 1977; **301**: 579–92.
2 Opie LH. Long distance running and sudden death. *N Engl J Med* 1975; **293**: 941–2.
3 Northcote R, Ballantyne D. Sudden cardiac death in sport. *BMJ* 1983; **287**: 1357–9.
4 Nicholl JP, Coleman P, Williams BT. The epidemiology of sports and exercise related injury in the United Kingdom. *Br J Sports Med* 1995; **29**: 232–8.
5 van Camp SP, Bloor CM, Mueller PO *et al*. Non-traumatic sports death in high school and college athletes. *Med Sci Sports Exer* 1995; **27**: 641–7.
6 Siscovick DS, Weiss NS, Fletcher RH, Lasky T. The incidence of primary cardiac arrest during vigorous exercise. *N Engl J Med* 1984; **311**: 874-7.
7 Thompson PD, Funk EJ, Carleton RA, Sturners WQ. Incidence of death during jogging in Rhode Island from 1975 through 1980. *JAMA* 1982; **247**: 2535–8.
8 Maron BJ, Shirani J, Poliac LC *et al*. Sudden death in young competitive athletes. *JAMA* 1996; **276**: 199–204.
9 Cantwell JD, Fontanarosa PB. An Olympic Medical Legacy. *JAMA* 1996; **276**: 248–9.
10 Weidenberger EJ, Krauss MD, Waller BF *et al*. Incorporation of the screening medical examination in the preparticipation exam. *Clin J Sports Med* 1995; **5**: 86–9.
11 Murray P, Cantwell JD, Heath D *et al*. The role of limited echocardiography in screening athletes. *Am J Cardiol* 1995; **76**: 849–50.
12 Fuller CM, McNulty CM, Spring DA *et al*. Prospective screening of 5,615 high school athletes for risk of sudden cardiac death. *Med Sci Sports Exer* 1997; **29**: 1131–8.
13 Bethesda Conference Report. 26th Bethesda Conference: Recommendations for determining eligibility for competition in athletes with cardiovascular abnormalities. Chaired by Maron BJ, Mitchell JH. *J Am Coll Cardiol* 1994; **24**: 848–99.
14 Thompson PD. The cardiovascular complications of vigorous physical activity. *Arch Intern Med* 1996; **156**: 2297–2302.
15 Ragosta M, Crabtree J, Sturner WQ, Thompson PD. Death during recreational exercise in the state of Rhode island. *Med Sci Sports Exerc* 1984; **16**: 339–42.
16 Toffler GH, Mittleman MA, Muller JE. Physical activity and the triggering of myocardial infarction: the case for regular exercise. *Heart* 1996; **75**: 323–5.

17 Mehta J, Mehta P, Horalek C. The significance of platelet vessel wall prostaglandin equilibrium during exercise induced stress. *Am Heart J* 1983; **105**: 895–900.
18 Khann PK, Seth HN, Balasubramanian V, Hoon RS. Effect of submaximal exercise on fibrinolytic activity in ischaemic heart disease. *BMJ* 1975; **ii**: 910–2.
19 Toffler GH, Stone PH, Maclure M *et al*. Analysis of possible triggers of acute myocardial infarction. *Am J Cardiol* 1990; **66**: 22–7.
20 Mittleman MA, Maclure M, Tofler GH *et al*. Triggering of acute myocardial infarction by heavy physical exertion. Protection against triggering by regular exertion. Determinants of the Myocardial Infarction Onset Study Investigators. *N Engl J Med* 1993; **329**: 1677–83.
21 American Heart Association Medical/Scientific Statement. Cardiac rehabilitation programmes. *Circulation* 1994; **90**: 1602–10.
22 Murray PM, Herrington DM, Pettus CW *et al*. Should patients with heart disease exercise in the morning or afternoon? *Arch Intern Med* 1993; **153**: 833–6.
23 Goble AJ, Hare DL, Macdonald PS *et al*. Effects of early programmes of high and low intensity exercise on physical performance after transmural acute myocardial infarction. *Br Heart J* 1991; **65**: 126–31.
24 Thompson PD, Klocke FJ, Levine BD, Vancamp SP. American College of Cardiology. Task Force 5. Coronary artery disease. *J Am Coll Cardiol* 1994; **24**: 888–92.
25 Henschen S, Skilanglauf and Skiwettlauf: Eine medizinische Sportstudie. *Mitt Klein* 1899; **2**: 15.
26 Sechtem U. The athlete's heart revisited. *Eur Heart J* 1996; **17**: 1138–40.
27 American Heart Association. Cardiovascular Preparticipation Screening of Competitive Athletes. *Med Sci Sports Exer* 1996; **28**: 1445–52.
28 Maron BJ *et al*. Risk profiles and cardiovascular preparticipation screening of competitive athletes. *Cardiol Clin* 1997; **15**: 473–83.
29 Maron BJ, Isner JM, McKenna WJ. 26th Bethesda Conference: recommendations for determining eligibility for competition in athletes with cardiovascular abnormalities. Task Force 3: hypertrophic cardiomyopathy, myocarditis and other myopericardial diseases and mitral valve prolapse. *J Am Coll Cardiol* 1994; **24**: 880–85.

9 Head injury

Concussion means brain damage even if only temporary; it is important not to underestimate its severity. The concussed athlete should not continue in the game, event or race because although their injury may be temporary and minor, they may have some subtle impairment of coordination or proprioception. As a result they may be more likely to injure themselves or others. If playing a contact sport, such loss of function may lead to injury in others, or if riding in a horse race, bike race or motor sport, any loss of judgement or coordination may lead to catastrophe.

The serious effects of head injury may not be immediately obvious and there are key rules to observe after any significant head injury. An athlete should not drink alcohol. The effects of alcohol make it impossible to detect minor loss of coordination in the early stages of intracranial haemorrhage. The player should be accompanied home and relatives informed: if knocked out, suffering from headaches, double vision or vomiting the patient should attend hospital.

Head injury in a sporting context can be devastating. It may be rare but the long-term sequelae in a young person and its cascade affect many members of a family. Boxing has attracted considerable adverse publicity and a number of high profile competitors have been involved in events that resulted in serious head injury and sometimes death. It is impossible to prevent serious head injury in a sport where the aim is to inflict punishment and where blows to the head form an integral part of the game. Serious head injury can occur in other sports too and it may be unfair to single out boxing when motor racing, rugby and horse racing are also exceedingly dangerous. Serious injury can rarely be prevented; doctors involved in sport should be acutely aware of the nature of presentation and important factors to consider in the event of such an injury.

Head injury prevention and head protection

In a sport such as boxing, the single blow is only part of the problem. Boxers hone their skill to deliver not just a direct blow, but to include a rotational force which increases the effect of the impact. Boxing injury is not caused simply by the impact alone but by the contrecoup injury. Head protection in boxers is therefore unlikely to reduce the devastating effect of a single direct blow with its additional rotational force as it strikes the chin. It may, however, reduce cuts and protect against eye injury. In severe acceleration or deceleration the brain, which is soft, is forced against the wall of the skull. The effect of a punch on the brain within the skull has been vividly described as of similar effect to vigorously shaking a jelly in a biscuit box. Such a blow causes both local bruising and more diffuse injury. The result of a cumulative series of blows causing minor injury can be more sinister and we can appreciate how recurrent minor injury producing laminar and oblique forces may rupture the smaller blood vessels in the cerebral cortex and can disrupt the networks of nerve links that make up the brain tissue.

Head protection can offer limited protection in other sports. The cycling helmet for example can offer some protection. They are tested for direct impact and most are only of value at speeds of less than 15 m.p.h. They do offer some protection but are inadequate at high speed where one would need a level of protection similar to that offered by a full face motor cycle helmet. This level of protection would clearly be impractical. In cricket, hockey and hurling the helmet offers protection principally in protecting against eye and facial injury. Only a severe blow will fracture the skull but serious head injury can occur in the absence of any bony injury.

Prehospital care in head injury

Prehospital emergency care can make a huge difference to morbidity. The priority, in the event of a serious injury, is to ensure brain oxygen perfusion and prevent secondary damage. It is often impossible to be certain that the patient has not also sustained a serious neck injury. For this reason, the casualty must be treated as if they have also had a neck injury. First aid measures should be applied using the ABC of emergency care. The airway is the priority. If medical equipment is available, oxygen should be delivered and in severe loss of consciousness it may be necessary to intubate the patient. Intravenous access through a drip will ensure that the patient does not become shocked, especially in the event of intra-abdominal trauma or limb fractures. Ideally blood pressure and pulse should be monitored although changes may be greatly delayed in a fit athlete.

Proper early management should prevent a second injury from brain ischaemia. This can occur due to obstruction of the airway or at the cellular level where local oedema obstructs microcirculation. If there has been an intracranial injury with ruptured blood vessels within the closed skull, the resulting haematoma will compress brain tissue. The only effective treatment of intracranial haematoma is evacuation, best undertaken at a specialist centre. After surgery there should be a reduction in oedema and resolution of symptoms. The greatest improvement occurs in the first week, although improvement may continue for some months.

The baseline neurological status should be established and monitored to pick up any deterioration. This can be done using the Glasgow coma scale, a system that may be used even by those with very basic knowledge. The key to proper management is to establish an airway, ensure oxygenation, maintain circulation and transport the patient to a neurosurgical centre as soon as possible.

Glasgow Coma Scale

Eye opening		Spontaneous	4
		To speech	3
		To pain	2
		No response	1
Best motor response	To verbal command		6
	To painful stimulus		
		Localises pain	5
		Flexion/withdrawal	4
		Flexion/abnormal	3
		Extension	2
		No response	1
Best verbal response		Oriented	5
		Confused	4
		Inappropriate words	3
		Incomprehensible sounds	2
		None	1
Total			3–15

Concussion

Concussion can be of variable severity [1]. After a minor injury there may be slight confusion but no loss of memory. With more severe injury there is confusion with retrograde amnesia. With severe head injury there is a classic postconcussion syndrome with transient unconsciousness, retrograde amnesia and significant post-traumatic amnesia. Retrograde amnesia is a loss of memory of events before the head injury and post-traumatic amnesia is loss of memory of events that happened after the injury. Severe head injury may lead to longer term problems which present in general practice. These include intermittent headaches and poor concentration which can last for some months.

Severity of concussion

Grade	Loss of consciousness	Post-traumatic amnesia
Mild	None	<30 min
Moderate	<5 min	>30 min
Severe	>5 min	>24 hr

Players may not wish to reveal that they have sustained a head injury to the medical officer at a match or in charge of a team in order to avoid a mandatory period of rest. Sports such as boxing, rugby and horse racing have guidelines which may prohibit participation for a period of time after an injury. If this is the case, and the athlete may lose money or status, they may be unwilling to reveal that they have sustained an injury. There is an important place in these sports for health promotion and advice about the nature of injury. Return to sport is always a contentious issue.

After head injury, the serious effects may not be immediately obvious. The evolution of a subdural haemorrhage may take some time and early signs can be easily missed. After a head injury it is important not to drink alcohol because the early signs of a more serious head injury may be masked by the effects of alcohol. The athlete who sustains such an injury should be accompanied home and relatives informed. They should also be told what to look out for. If knocked out or suffering from headache, double vision or vomiting the patient should be brought to hospital. This information should be given to the patient and their escort, preferably on a printed card such as the example shown here.

Head injury advice

You have just attended hospital and the medical staff have found no evidence of a serious head injury. From now on there should be a gradual improvement in your condition. In the next 24 hours you should not consume alcohol, drive a car or use any dangerous machinery and you should always have someone with you. If you, or whoever is with you, notices any of the following problems you should return to hospital immediately:

- If you are difficult to rouse
- Vomiting (more than once)
- Severe or increasing headache, dizziness, drowsiness or double vision.

Reference

1 Harries M, Williams C, Stanish WD, Micheli LJ. *The Oxford Textbook of Sports Medicine*. Oxford Medical Publications, 1996.

10 Spine and neck injury

Spinal injuries do occur and the sequelae of such injuries are devastating. Depending on the level and extent of the injury, partial or complete paralysis may occur. Although the primary aim must be to avoid such injury, if serious accidents do occur we must ensure there is no further damage. The sports doctor should be familiar with neck collars and how to measure the correct size and apply them. They should also be able to put on splints, fracture pads and apply slings and bandages.

Cervical spine injury

Acute cervical spine injuries are rare in general practice but the team doctor or event doctor may be asked to treat a suspected cervical spine injury. Cervical spine injury is most common in high speed trauma but can occur in many sports including horse riding, rugby football, skiing and diving. Accidental injury is well documented in those who dive mistakenly into partially filled or empty pools. From a general practice perspective immediate care is the most critical because of the devastating potential sequelae of mismanagement.

If the injury occurs in a contact or combat sport, the match should be stopped as soon as the injury occurs and medical personnel should take control. It is most important to have a high index of suspicion and treat any neck injury as potentially serious. The doctor should stay with the patient and have an ambulance requested, asking specifically for a scoop stretcher. If the patient is unconscious, maintenance of the airway and neck stabilisation are the priority. If the patient is to be moved onto their back this should only be undertaken using a proper 'log roll' technique. If a collar is available, the correct size collar should be applied. The patient should not be moved so the event must be stopped until the patient is removed by ambulance.

The surgical or conservative management and rehabilitation are a matter for the specialists. Occasionally, X-rays taken at screening or medical examination reveal congenital abnormalities including those of the atlanto–axial joint. The athlete should be excluded from sport until specialist opinion is sought. The management may include stabilisation, in which case endurance type sports may be permitted but contact sports should be prohibited for life.

Back pain

Back pain in the athlete is a diagnostic challenge. Diagnosis is difficult, sometimes impossible, and treatment can be slow and frustrating. Back pain can ruin a sports career and at times both athlete and physician feel powerless. It constitutes about 10% of all athletic injuries. The most common causes include disc lesions, spondylosis (which is more common in particular sports) and postural back pain which may be due not so much to posture but to the rather extreme training regimes and biomechanical stress of top-class sport. Teamwork is the key to management and should include the athlete, coach and physiotherapist.

Features of the pain may suggest a diagnosis. A standard medical history will reveal details of the site, nature, duration and radiation of the pain. Night pain suggests a sinister cause and demands urgent attention. The character of the pain may also help as a muscular pain is often described as a spasm, aching describes skeletal pain, and radiating pain suggests neurological involvement. Radiating pain may be further described in the classic pattern associated with one or more nerve roots. Spinal stenosis is associated with exertion-type pain with the trunk extended as in running or walking and is relieved on sitting where the spine is flexed. Cycling or rowing, for example, seldom cause this pain. Other non-sporting causes of pain include arthritis, where the pain is worse in the morning and eases through the day.

Back examination

Inspection

Look for general muscular development. Look for symmetry with level shoulders, a straight spine and level iliac crests. Alterations in the posture may be due to skeletal abnormalities such as leg length discrepancy causing asymmetry of the iliac crests and compensatory scoliosis. In some back injuries there may be an apparent scoliosis due to muscular spasm.

Active movement

Flexion, extension, lateral flexion and rotation. One may record the degree of flexion by how far the finger tips can extend in relation to the legs. For example to the knee, mid-tibia, ankle etc. If you wish to record flexion accurately you may use a goniometer. It is important to identify where the flexion occurs and if there is free movement of all the vertebrae. With flexion we can also look to see if any apparent scoliosis disappears. Pain may occur during flexion and the relationship of the pain to flexion may give useful clues to the site and nature of the problem. Forward flexion causes anterior pressure on the vertebral and intervertebral discs so that pain on flexion may be due to a disc lesion. Extension stresses the posterior structures including the pars interarticularis and facet joints so that pain on extension may suggest spondylolysis or facet joint problems. Palpation of the back should include palpation of the spinous processes and the sacral area. The patient should now be examined on the couch, and important information can be gleaned from observing the patient climb onto the couch.

Specific examination

While supine the physician may examine straight leg raising, recording the appropriate angle. One should also examine hamstring flexibility as this may indicate the cause of the limited straight leg raising and as it is commonly associated with spondylolysis. The hips should be examined for flexion and internal and external rotation. There should be an assessment of the sacroiliac joints by squeezing the pelvis at the iliac crests. A neurological examination should include examination for loss of sensation and testing the reflexes at the knee and ankle.

The Slump test is a more effective method of assessing for nerve root pain. Finally, the one legged hyperextension test is a diagnostic test for spondylolysis which may be due to pars interarticularis fracture.

Back pain is a common problem in the normal practice population and the majority of patients suffer from back pain at some time in their lives. The guidelines from the Royal College of Radiologists suggest that X-ray is not an appropriate first line investigation with back pain. The situation is rather different in the keen athlete where speed of investigation and treatment is critical. If the clinical signs suggest spondylolysis it is important to ask for oblique views which can better demonstrate the pars interarticularis fracture. If nerve root compression is suspected, the CAT scan is the most appropriate first line radiographic investigation. Routine blood tests should also be undertaken. In the absences of radiographic cause referral to a specialist is appropriate for further investigation with bone scan.

Management of acute back injury

The acronym TREAT for treatment, rehabilitation, exercise, activity and target, is a useful *aide-memoire* for management of various sports injuries.

Treatment
Acute back injuries must be treated as an emergency. The back should be stabilised and the patient transported to hospital. There is no place for first aid intervention other than maintenance of an airway and stabilisation. A simple musculoskeletal injury that does not require investigation or specialist treatment may progress to the next stage.

Rehabilitation
Mobilisation is the first stage in rehabilitation. Traction may be used for pain relief in disc lesions as it can help separate the vertebral bodies. Gentle manipulation can help in the early stages but is limited by pain. Manipulation is usually by gentle rhythmic movement. Massage is useful in pain relief and in reducing muscle spasm. Resume muscle activity with isometric strengthening initially. This can be done by pushing against a fixed surface such as a wall. Physiotherapists may use heat, massage and various electrical treatments.

Exercise
Having achieved the first phase of rehabilitation the next stage is to begin progressive dynamic exercises to improve spinal posture and to move on to exercises such as swimming initially and later

to jogging, running and cycling. One may also begin strengthening exercises and continue with stretching.

Activity
The next stage is the beginning of sport-specific activity. While the previous phase concentrated on non-specific activity this phase is about getting back to all the movements associated with the sport.

Target
The target is the return to competitive sport. It is essential to include a preventative strategy to avoid recurrence of the injury. The athlete and coach should look closely at any precipitating factors in the sport or equipment. The athlete should perform a pre-activity warm-up, stretching, and warm-down together with an exercise programme to strengthen both agonists and antagonists. This means both abdominal and back strengthening exercises.

Management of chronic back pain

Back pain may be due to a disc lesion. Referred pain is not always present and the diagnosis may not be immediately clear from the history and examination. The initial treatment is rest and symptomatic management. Sport is avoided and should only be attempted when there is full pain-free range of movement and should be preceded by a progressive rehabilitation programme supervised by a physiotherapist. In most cases surgery is the last option but there is often considerable pressure on the physician to do something. The neurosurgical approach is recommended.

Spondylolysis is a frustrating problem for the athlete. It is often a low grade backache which is worse with sport, but seems not to cause problems away from sport. Indeed, skeletal surveys have shown a remarkably high prevalence of asymptomatic spondylosis in the non-athletic population. The problem is a fracture of the pars interarticularis which seems to be a stress-related fracture due to repeated hyperextension. It may be obvious on an oblique X-ray, although in the early stages plain X-ray may not show the defect and it may only be demonstrated using bone scan or on CAT scan. It is important to try to identify these lesions early to ensure that the stress injury does not become a complete fracture and modify exercise or begin bracing early. The longer a fracture remains, the less likely it is to respond to conservative management. If this lesion is identified then specialist opinion is required to define the next line of management, but rest is a key feature. If the fracture is recent, some specialists recommend immobilisation using a plaster jacket or brace but return to sport is unlikely for at least 6 months. In failure of conservative management surgery may be necessary but draws the risk of complications including loss of lumbar motion and transmission of additional stress on neighbouring vertebrae and subsequent stress fractures.

The physical stress of the sport can lead to a mechanical back pain. The diagnosis is one of exclusion, when all investigations including X-ray, and CAT scan are negative. Two sports in which mechanical back pain are common include rowing and cycling. Both sports put similar stress of the low back with explosive leg extension from a flexed position. Training for rowing tends to mimic the activities in the boat and heavy resistance training may be undertaken using weight exercises with leg flexion and an unsupported lower spine. Changes in the type of blade on oars has led to a similar problem where the lower back is asked to brace against a sudden leg extension against large resistance. Tired muscles cannot completely protect the ligaments of the lower spine with resulting backache. Cycling can cause similar problems. In fact, backache is a problem experienced by many cyclists from the modest veteran to the top professionals. This is a nagging low backache that comes on during a long ride, in a race, or in training. It is partly due to the ergonomically unsound cycling position with the back held horizontal over the top tube, the neck hyperextended and the knee fully flexed during the pedal stroke. The long periods spent training and racing in this position stress the ligaments of the lower spine, especially when the muscles are tired after a long hard ride. In most cycle races there are periods of relative calm which allow the cyclist to change their posture, stand on the pedals and stretch. The pressure on the lower back with each pedal rotation can be reduced by the technique of spinning, where experienced cyclists use a high cadence and low gear. This reduces the pressure with each pedal rotation and reduces the pressure on the lower back. It also helps to improve the flexibility of the lower back. In addition, the abdominal muscles in cyclists are notoriously lax and cannot help stabilise the back. Cyclists should therefore undertake general training to ensure that they have good muscle tone. The older cyclist is often not as well able to spin and may rely more on high gears. Together with reduced flexibility and perhaps some arthritic changes in the lumbar spine, chronic ligament pain can be more of a problem. The mature cyclist with backache should also look at other aspects of lifestyle which make back pain worse, including techniques of lifting, spending long periods in the car and the posture adopted at work. It also helps to raise the handlebars relative to the saddle as what is lost in aerodynamics may be gained in comfort.

Sports such as gymnastics and activities like dance which require hyperlordosis and rapid flexion and extension are more likely to produce spondylolysis. These are essentially overuse injuries associated with the typical movements of the sport. Backache in these athletes demands a high index of suspicion and X-ray assessment. Prevention strategies should include a variation in the training routines in an effort to reduce overuse, padded landing areas and well cushioned landing pits. Other sports where hyperextension forms an integral part of the sport include athletic events such as the pole vault, high jump, the butterfly stroke in swimming, most lifts in weight lifting and forced hyperextension occurs in the tackle in contact sports such as American Football and both codes of rugby football. Rotational sports such as golf, cricket and tennis are more likely to cause intervertebral disc problems.

Managing chronic back pain in non-athletes is not easy in general practice. While bed rest was advised in the past, early activity within the limit of pain is now the treatment of choice. Rest may exacerbate back pain in some people and certainly delays recovery. Physical activity, however strange this may sound, is recommended [1]. The type of activity does not appear to be important, providing that it does not cause pain. It has been suggested [2] that the mechanism for improvement in symptoms, although still unclear, is a reduction of the oedema and venous congestion that occurs around the nerve roots in the vertebral canal and intervertebral foramen. The reduction of symptoms may, however, be due to inhibition of the pain signal through either muscle activity or joint movement. In any event, those with back pain are advised to undertake gentle exercise within the limits of pain.

Back problems in children

The causes of back pain tend to be different in young adults. In one study [3] of adolescent athletes presenting with back pain, 47% were found to have a spondylolysis stress fracture of the pars interarticularis compared to 5% of adult controls. Only 11% of the adolescents had discogenic back pain compared to 48% of the adults. Only 6% of the adolescents had musculotendinous problems while this was much more a problem in adults where it accounted for 27% of cases. No problems with spinal stenosis were found in the adolescents yet this occurred in 10% of adults. Excessive lumbar lordosis may occur during the adolescent growth spurt. This can give rise to low back pain. There is rarely any serious pathological condition and the appropriate treatment is to encourage exercises to increase hamstring and low back flexibility. They can usually continue in sport.

Scheuermann's disease

In Scheuermann's disease there is kyphosis of the thoracic spine in adolescence. The diagnosis is made when there are three or more adjoining vertebrae with 5° or more of wedging. There may be disc narrowing and changes to the end plates with Schmorls nodes. It may give back pain, but the most common findings are of a rounded back and tight hamstrings. It is usually not a contra-indication to sport. If there are symptoms of pain the treatment is rest and occasionally bracing. Scoliosis requires specialist referral.

Back pain in sport: summary

- Back pain in the sports person is different from back pain in the general population
- Investigation should be early and include X-ray: anterior, lateral and oblique
- CAT scan and bone scan may be needed early
- Spondylolysis is common in children.

References

1 Clinical Standards Advisory Group. *Back pain*. London, HMSO, 1994.
2 Jayson MIV. Physical activity is best for back pain. *BMJ* 1997; **315**: 771.
3 Michaeli L, Wood R. Back pain in young athletes. *Arch Pediatr Adolesc Med* 1995; **149**: 15–18.

11 Injuries of the upper limb

Many sports injuries occur at the shoulder. These may be loosely classified into those associated with trauma and those associated with overuse. The general practitioner's interest in trauma management usually begins when the athlete is discharged from the accident and emergency department or fracture clinic and visits the surgery for advice on rehabilitation and return to sport. In contrast, however, is the frequent presentation of overuse and chronic shoulder pain. Those who act as team medical officer or touchline doctor will encounter traumatic shoulder injuries. One of the most common, and indeed one of the most important roles of the general practitioner is in advice on rehabilitation after a dislocated shoulder.

Examination of the shoulder

This is a simple guide and not intended to be a substitute for a comprehensive description of examination technique. Its purpose is to act as a reminder to GPs who have already learned the technique, but have stored it deep in the recesses of their mind.

Inspection

Look for swelling, and the contours of the shoulder and neck. In particular look for abnormal appearance, including steps in the clavicle or excessive mobility of the distal end of the clavicle. Look also at muscle definition and for wasting.

Active movements

Examine all the movements of the shoulder: flexion, extension, abduction, adduction and rotation. This sequence of examination may help.

Ask the patient to place their hands by their sides and to lift the arms laterally above their head and join hands in the middle. This simple movement, observed from the front and behind, can demonstrate many of the possible problems associated with the shoulder. Look in particular for smooth abduction. Three key abnormalities to look for are: problems with the supraspinatus where the patient uses a hitching movement to abduct the shoulder the first 15° before the deltoid can take over; a painful arc in the middle range of movement, from 60° to 120°, which may occur with supraspinatus tendinitis or subacromial bursitis and no movement above the horizontal, which may occur with a capsulitis or frozen shoulder. With adhesive capsulitis, there is no glenohumeral movement so that any shoulder movement occurs at the scapula. There is some abduction at the scapula but the patient can only bring the arm to the horizontal by hunching the shoulder. This scapular movement, in the absence of any gleno-humeral movement, is best seen from behind.

Problems with the other components of the rotator cuff may have already been spotted as the patient tries to take off their jacket or shirt before examination. With limitation of external rotation, the patient takes off the sleeve of the contralateral side first. On examination one should look for limitation of internal and external rotation. Ask the patient to place their arm in the neutral position, with the elbow flexed, and then rotate the arm inwards and outward. It is usually easiest you do these movements yourself and to ask the patient to copy you. Alternatively, these movements may be assessed in a more functional way by asking the patient to scratch their back, as high up as they can (to assess internal rotation) and to put their hand behind their neck and scratch down as far as they can (external rotation). Passive movements are of relatively little value.

Palpation

Palpate the surface anatomy along the spine of the scapula to the acromium, for the coracoid process and along the clavicle. Feel for the stability of the clavicle.

Resisted movements

Simply resist the flexion, extension, abduction, adduction and rotational shoulder movements.

Special tests

With the supraspinatus injury, resisted abduction in the middle range of movement is weak. The impingement sign may also be positive.

The apprehension test for recurrent dislocation of the shoulder mimics the movement that causes dislocation. To do this test, relax the patient, usually lying supine, flex the elbow and abduct the shoulder so the arm is horizontal. If you now attempt to externally rotate the shoulder the patient may not allow you as they sense the instability and are, as the test suggests, apprehensive. There are other shoulder instability tests, including the drawer sign, but these are more for the specialists.

There are other tests for the shoulder which can be used by those with experience and expertise. These include the tests for dislocation, the sulcus sign, and the drawer test. Yergason's test is for the bicipital tendon.

Dislocation of the shoulder

Shoulder dislocation is usually reduced in the Accident and Emergency Department. Some sports doctors will reduce dislocations on the field of play but this introduces a number of diagnostic and possible medicolegal complications. On the other hand, some athletes have recurrent dislocations, they know exactly what has happened when their shoulder pops out, and immediate reduction may be justified.

In most cases, after reduction of the shoulder, the joint is immobilised. This allows the pain and swelling to reduce and early repair of the soft tissues to begin to repair. The capsule will be stretched, there may be some damage to the rotator cuff and the labrum may have been torn. For 2 weeks the patient has the shoulder strapped close to the trunk. Recurrent dislocations of the shoulder are very common, and the athlete must not try to accelerate this early phase of treatment. After two weeks they begin a planned rehabilitation and strengthening programme, closely monitored by a physiotherapist so there is no excessive abduction of the shoulder. After a further 2 weeks (4 weeks since the injury) they may begin to increase the range of movement and vary the resistance exercises. It is essential to stick closely to this plan. There is no long-term gain in trying to accelerate the process as recurrent dislocation have a major impact on a sporting career.

Shoulder examination checklist

Inspection
- front and behind
- look for muscle wasting

Palpation
- clavicle
- bony landmarks

Movements
- functional
- hands above head
- glenohumeral
- hands up the back
- hands down the back

Anatomical movements
- abduction, adduction
- flexion, extension
- internal and external rotation

Apprehension test
Drawer sign
Impingement sign
Winging of scapula

Fracture of the clavicle

It is rare to realign a fracture of the clavicle and in most cases the injury is allowed to heal regardless of the aesthetic appearance. For most athletes functional recovery is more important than appearance. The clavicle often heals with a visible step but the union is usually strong enough to withstand normal trauma. After attendance at Accident and Emergency and X-ray confirmation of the injury, the patient is sent home with collar and cuff. They may begin to mobilise the shoulder again in 2–3 weeks. Most fractures require about 6 weeks to achieve good bony union. Likewise with the collar bone. This does not mean, however, that an athlete cannot do any training. For the first 2 weeks the shoulder will be too painful to do much movement. After about 2 weeks the fracture will have some stability, as fibrous tissue and some organisation occurs across the fracture site. Although not nearly as strong as bone it is moderately stable and the patient may begin to do some active work, cycling on a stationary bicycle for example. As recovery progresses, the shoulder will become more stable, less painful, and some training is possible. In 4–6 weeks the athlete can return to aerobic activities, swimming and running, but contact sports take a further 2 weeks.

Dislocation of the acromio–clavicular joint is a common injury especially in contact sports but in most cases requires no treatment other than rest. The injury heals but often, because of rupture of the acromio–clavicular ligaments, the distal end of the clavicle is left mobile and floating. It is possible in many cases to press on the clavicle and feel it move up and down freely on its ligament. Although some suggest complex strapping arrangements to treat these injuries, this strapping is usually useless.

Rotator cuff injuries

The rotator cuff muscles surround the shoulder joint and blend in with the capsule. There are four main muscles: supraspinatus, infraspinatus, subscapularis and teres minor. For those who cannot remember their anatomy, the names of these muscles give it away. After first locating the spine of the scapula, it is easy to identify the position of the supraspinatus above the spine, the infraspinatus, below and the subscabular is under the scapula and anterior. Teres minor is a little more obscure but lies below the infraspinatus. Knowing a little of the anatomy, it is easy to understand the functional tests of the shoulder joint (Figure 11.1).

Overuse injuries of the shoulder are common especially in throwing or racket sports. These injuries are easily seen on MRI, which at times reveal other associated injuries. Rotator cuff injuries require intensive treatment usually with physiotherapy and progressive rehabilitation and the muscles of the

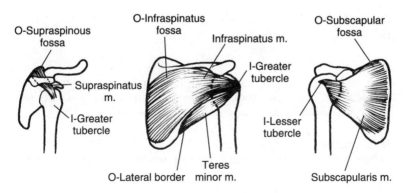

Figure 11.1 The rotator cuff muscles.

rotator cuff may be trained specifically bearing in mind their function.

Supraspinatus tendinitis is one of the most common chronic injuries. It may be accompanied by subacromial bursitis. This is an impingement injury and often occurs due to the action of the supraspinatus in the subacromial space. With inflammation in the tendon or in the bursa, the pain occurs when the subacromial tissue is squeezed in overarm movements. The diagnostic test is the impingement test: flex the elbow and the shoulder holding them at 90° to the vertical. The forearm should now be held across the chest. Internally rotate the shoulder by dropping the forearm and which brings the greater diameter of the head of humerus into the subacromial space. This causes an impingement of the supraspinatus tendon or bursa in the subacromial space and is painful if they are inflammed. Ultrasound and muscle retraining can help but an injection is often needed.

Injection of the shoulder joint

The lateral approach to inject the shoulder joint injection is easiest. You can identify the acromium from the surface anatomy. Insert the needle below the acromium, aiming medial and upwards, as if aiming for the ear. There should be an easy passage into the joint and the injection should meet no resistance (Figure 11.2). Inject only if there is no resistance as we ought never to inject into a tendon.

Management of shoulder injury

Remember the acronym for management of injuries: TREAT for treatment, rehabilitation, exercise, activity and target.

Treatment
Rest and ice are applied at first. Non-steroidal anti-inflammatory medication can help reduce pain and inflammation. Physiotherapy should be early and include ultrasound.

Rehabilitation
When pain-free, the patient should begin stretching exercises for abduction, flexion and extension, and internal and external rotation. Muscle strengthening is begun with gentle isometric strengthening initially. This can be done by contracting the

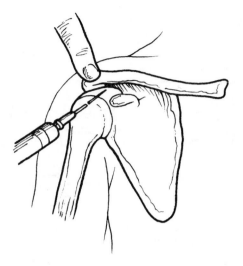

Figure 11.2 Injection of subacromial bursa in the shoulder.

muscle against a fixed surface. Later isotonic exercise may be included using rolls of elastic cord or cliniband (Figure 11.3). Physiotherapists may use heat, massage and various electrical treatments.

Exercise

The next stage is progressive dynamic movement: abduction, adduction, and internal and external rotation in particular. The patient should also continue with stretching.

Activity

Next comes the beginning of sport-specific movement, with a gradual and progressive return to sport-specific exercise. While the previous phase concentrated on general activity this phase is about getting back to all the movements associated with the sport. Overarm movements can be introduced, initially slower and with reduced resistance.

Target

The target is a return to competitive sport, but it is essential to include a preventive strategy to avoid recurrence of the injury. If there is pain the athlete must stop and return to first principles.

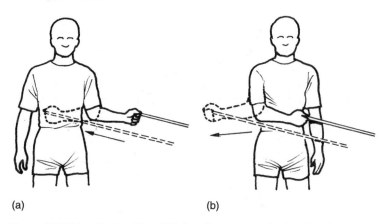

(a)   (b)

Figure 11.3 Using elastic tubing (Cliniband) to exercise the shoulder: (a) stretching the subscapularis muscle and (b) stretching the infraspinatus and teres minor muscles.

Tennis elbow (lateral epicondylitis)

Tennis elbow causes pain at the lateral epicondyle. It is a nagging pain, often described as being like a toothache. It is not always due to sport and may be associated with any repetitive activity of the extensor muscles of the forearm. It takes the name tennis elbow because it is frequently associated with the backhand stroke in tennis. The pain is worse on extension of the arm, on lifting a heavy object, on gripping, making a fist and on shaking hands. While the point of tenderness is on the lateral eipcondyle, the pain may be a shooting pain radiating down the forearm or up into the upper arm.

It is an apophysitis or traction overuse injury where the extensor muscles arise at the common extensor origin on the lateral epicondyle. Treatment is aimed at both symptomatic management and treating the cause which means reducing the forces applied to the extensor mechanism. Symptomatic treatment includes ice. An icepack can be applied for 20–30 minutes every 4–6 hours for a number of days until the pain eases. It is also possible to massage the injury site with ice. A very effective method of making your own cold applicator is to freeze some water in a paper cup and then tear away the top part of the cup, leaving an ideal ice applicator. Ice can be massaged onto the tender area for 5–10 minutes. It is, of course, important in the application of any ice therapy to ensure that the skin is not burned by the ice. Anti-inflammatory medication, either in tablet form or as a topical treatment, is also of benefit.

Treating the cause means reducing or altering the force causing the injury. For example, where it is caused by tennis this may include altering the technique to reduce the jarring impact on the backhand stroke, by altering the size of the racket, or avoiding playing in damp weather outdoors when the tennis balls may be slightly heavier. It is also possible to modify both the impact and the direction of traction using a forearm brace or tennis elbow strap which can be bought in sport and medical retail outlets. This strap wraps firmly around the forearm constricting the extensor muscles just distal to the lateral epicondyle. This can alter the direction of traction and reduces the direct force on the tendon origin.

Physiotherapy using friction massage and ultrasound can be of benefit. Even with treatment the condition may persist and it may be necessary to have a period of complete rest from the causative activity.

Injection of tennis elbow

If conservative management of tennis elbow is ineffective, corticosteroid injection may be helpful. The usual dose is about 2–5 ml of a short-acting corticosteroid such as hydrocortisone acetate. Doctors worry about possible side-effects of corticosteroid injections and in most cases our major concern is of local tissue degeneration due the catabolic effect on collagen. With tennis elbow this is less of a worry as surgical treatment of tennis elbow is by release of the origin and any possible rupture of fibres of the origin has the same overall outcome. By convention however, three injections only are given. Another possible side-effect of steroid injections is depigmentation and this is a realistic possibility in fit athletic people with minimal subcutaneous fat. The injection should be locally infiltrated around the area of maximum tenderness.

Tennis elbow can be a frustrating condition which comes and goes and, even when the symptoms have eased, return to sport may bring back the pain. While the aim of all treatment and rehabilitation is rapid return to activity, it is usual, in tennis elbow, to err on the side of caution. The time needed before return to sport is determined by the reduction of symptoms and speed of rehabilitation and not by the length of time since the onset of the injury. The return to sport should be very gradual and progressive. The patient may begin to play tennis gently when they can hold the racket firmly without pain, but full return should only be when there is full forearm strength and pain-free muscle contraction. If there is any pain the patient should stop the activity and begin a gradual progressive return.

Prevention of tennis elbow is technique- and equipment-related. Technical expertise and the use of the correct grip size helps reduce the problem. Exercises to improve flexion and extension strength, together with pronation and supination, can help.

Golfer's elbow

This is the traction apophysitis of the forearm flexors on the medial epicondyle. It takes its name from the forearm flexion that occurs when the golfer swings into the stroke. The management is similar, although most general practitioners are not so keen to inject medially due to the risk of damaging the ulnar nerve.

Injuries to the wrist

There are many potential injuries to the wrist. It is useful to know about these but in most cases they should be managed by an orthopaedic surgeon.

Fractures of the radius and ulna, including the Colles' and Smith's fracture, occur in many sports with a fall on the outstretched hand. The management of these injuries is no different from normal orthopaedic practice. A plaster cast is usually applied for about 6 weeks and thereafter specific rehabilitation depends on the nature of each individual sport. General fitness can be maintained through out.

The scaphoid fracture is common and, as we all know, requires particular attention. The scaphoid plaster makes maintenance of general fitness slightly more difficult.

Injuries to the small bones of the wrist are difficult to treat and require orthopaedic expertise. Common dislocations include dislocation of the lunate or the capitate. The hook of hamate can be injured by direct trauma, such as may occur in racket sports, hurling or hockey.

Tenovaginitis/tenosynovitis

Inflammation of the tendons of the forearm is common, especially in rowers where the repetitive rotation of the forearm with contraction of the flexors and extensors can cause inflammation of the tendons as they cross the medial side of the wrist. This is also known as de Quervain disease. Initially this causes an ache on exertion which may be progressive. It often occurs at the start of the season, after a period of rest, or with a sudden increase in training load. If a rower changes position so their oar is on the other side, known as 'changing sides' they must rotate (known as feathering) the oar with the other hand. This changes the movements of their wrists and may precipitate tenosynovitis. Initially there is pain but this may increase with swelling in the tendon sheath. There may be crepitus and the tendon sheath feels spongy. The first stage of treatment is rest to allow the inflammation to ease. Physiotherapy using ultrasound particularly helps reduce the inflammation. Anti-inflammatory gels help and injection into the tendon sheath is an option of last resort.

Finkelstein's test is used as an aid to diagnosis. Ask the athlete to make a fist with the thumb tucked inside. Ulnar deviation of the wrist will cause pain over the abductor pollicis longus and extensor pollicis brevis.

Common hand injuries

Skier's thumb

Winter brings a group of patients with thumb injuries to the surgery. They may have recently returned from a ski trip or from the artificial ski slope. The injury is an avulsion of the ulnar collateral ligament of the metacarpal phalangeal joint of the thumb. A torn ligament will leave considerable lateral laxity at the MCP joint. In many cases this injury is ignored. Some of these injuries heal but the ligament may not repair if it has slipped under the adductor aponeurosis. It is impossible to detect, on examination, if this has occurred. The surgical advice is for early repair, and if this could affect the patient's occupation it is certainly to be advised. An X-ray will indicate if a small fragment of bone has been avulsed. This makes management more clear cut and if the bone fragment is not displaced, it can be treated conservatively. The main message is that this seemingly minor injury can cause long-term instability and it is best to seek an expert orthopaedic opinion. This injury may occur in two ways, either due to the grip on the ski pole or from catching the thumb in the mesh of the artificial slope. It is a common injury and can be a major problem in those who need a fine grip at work. Skier's thumb may be preventable by gripping the ski pole without locking the ski pole tag with their thumb. Some skiers do not use the ski pole toggle at all. On an artificial slope, skiers should keep their arms close to their body and fists closed when they fall – easy to write, but difficult to do!

This injury is often confused with gamekeeper's thumb. In gamekeeper's thumb there is no ligament rupture, but the ligament has become stretched. It takes its name allegedly because gamekeepers stretched the ligament by breaking rabbit's necks!

Cyclists' numbness

Cyclists risk temporary neuropraxia of the ulnar nerve from pressure on the hands on the handlebars. In one major long distance cycling event, up to 20% recorded weakness of the hands, sufficient to cause difficulty holding a pen or a cup. Sensory symptoms were more common, affecting up to 40%. In most cases the symptoms were attributable to the ulnar nerve, although some had symptoms relating the the medial nerve and indeed some had both. This can occur because of the compression of the ulnar nerve at the hypothenar eminence. Symptoms usually ease after some days, but if the cyclist persists in spite of the injury, the resulting neuropraxia can give symptoms for many months.

Finger injury

Fractures, dislocations and ligamentous injuries are common in ball sports and contact sports. Finger dislocations can usually be reduced simply and splinted. It is important, however, to X-ray the finger to ensure that there is no bony damage. A damaged terminal phalanx or DIP joint can lead to long-term disability in those who need manual dexterity in their work. In most cases the injury can be treated most easily immediately after it occurs. Early management is best with later X-ray, unless a fracture is obvious. Fractures should be seen by an orthopaedic expert to ensure satisfactory functional recovery.

Mallet finger occurs when the extensor tendon is avulsed from the terminal phalanx. This occurs for example when the top of the finger is struck by a ball causing a sudden forced flexion. A small fragment of bone may also be avulsed. This injury is treated using a mallet finger splint for about 6 weeks. Players can continue to train in almost all aspect of the game, although clearly playing the sport itself can be difficult. Players tend to cheat and slip the splint off. This can lead to long-term deformity. Most other ligament injuries to the fingers require no more than strapping to the neighbouring finger.

12 Injuries of the abdomen, groin, hip and thigh

The sports doctor is most likely to encounter acute sports-related abdominal injuries when on the touchline at a contact sports event. The main concern with any acute abdominal injury is to exclude damage to the internal organs. The nature of any collision on the sports field is such that serious internal injury is unlikely, but if there is any doubt the patient should be referred to hospital. This is not the case in motor sport or even cycle racing: when the damage can be much more serious with a spectrum of injury similar to any acute trauma. A serious abdominal injury is a medical emergency.

Although serious intra-abdominal injury is unlikely the possibility must always be considered. The organs most susceptible are the spleen, liver and kidneys but these organs are well protected and unless there is previous damage should be relatively safe. One must be careful about the spleen because it may be damaged if it is enlarged and splenomegaly can occur in infectious mononucleosis. For this reason, players should not participate in contact sport when glandular fever is suspected. If glandular fever is confirmed they should only compete if there has been a negative abdominal ultrasound examination. Liver damage is also unlikely (unless there is hepatomegaly) because the liver is well protected. In the presence of a rib fracture, however, it is possible for a jagged fracture to penetrate the liver. Renal contusion can occur and the presence of haematuria requires serious consideration.

Genital trauma

Surprisingly, genital injuries are uncommon. Direct trauma may occur in contact sports, sometimes with lacerations requiring suture. In most cases of bruising the appropriate treatment is with ice (or cold), analgesia and scrotal support. Severe perineal injuries require specialist assessment as there may be ureter or prostate injury. Damage to the urethra occurs in front of the pelvic bones due to direct trauma. In pelvic fractures, the urethra may be damaged posteriorly. All meatal bleeding requires urgent hospital investigation. Those at risk in cricket or hockey should wear adequate protection.

In women the urethra is shorter and less vulnerable to direct trauma. Direct blows, such as falling on a beam, rarely cause urethral damage but may cause severe vulval bruising. An unusual but serious injury in women is vaginal douching that can occur in water skiing if the skier is wearing inadequate clothing. Women should always wear a wet suit with perineal protection. High pressure vaginal douche may cause vaginal wall trauma and infection, particularly salpingitis, may occur.

A common question asked by patients is if excessive cycling causes impotence. The evidence is that, among other hazards of long-distance cycling, impotence and numbness of the penis do occur. These symptoms are likely to be due to pressure on the pudendal nerve as it passes from the perineum to the skin of the penis and scrotum. Cyclists are advised to regularly change the position of the perineum on the saddle [1].

Haematuria

In practice we investigate unexplained haematuria. Exercise-induced haematuria and haemaglobinuria can occur with benign aetiology but this should be a diagnosis only after exclusion of serious pathology. Clearly after trauma in contact sport we are concerned about kidney damage. Hospital investigation is usually required and often admission is necessary. Kidney contusion requires close observation with bed rest. Investigation by IVP is recommended initially and further investigation is often required.

Haematuria can occur in runners without serious cause. The diagnosis is usually one of exclusion, but a running aetiology is always a differential diagnosis. It is thought to be due to bladder trauma as the bladder walls rub together with each step. One means of prevention is to ensure that the bladder is not empty when running.

Haemoglobinuria is a theoretical but rare condition. It is believed to be due to haemolysis following the trauma associated with recurrent foot strike in running. The likelihood is greatest the harder the foot strike and the longer the period spent running.

During the marathon boom, many people, totally unsuited to running, ran long distances. They were often overweight, wearing inadequate footwear, and foot impact was excessive.

The hip examination

The first component of hip is examination is in the observation of the patient walking. They may walk with a limp or irregular gait.

Inspection

Examine the position of the hips and the degree of anteversion. Examine also from the rear for asymmetry of the buttocks and skin creases. If there is any doubt about leg length this should be measured by tape measure from the anterior superior iliac spine to the medial malleolus.

Inspection is focused in particular on gait problems, apparent limb length discrepancy, bruising and swelling. In Trendelenberg's test the patient is asked to stand on one leg. Normally the pelvis on the other side should be slightly higher. If the other side drops this indicates either an unstable hip or weak hip abductors, i.e. the gluteus medius muscle.

Palpation

Most hip and thigh injuries are muscular so it is important to think of the quadriceps, hamstring and adductor muscle groups. Hip joint pain is usually felt at the groin crease. Trochanteric bursitis causes pain on the outer thigh over the greater trochanter. Other medical problems that may cause hip pain include lymphadenopathy, herniae and testicular problems including epididymitis. It may be appropriate to measure leg length.

Active, resisted and passive movements

When supine the patient should be asked to fully flex the hip. Extension can only be properly examined prone. For passive movements, flexion and rotation can be examined with the patient supine. Loss of hip movement is first noted in loss of internal rotation. Thomas' test is a test for hip movement including flexion and extension. The angle of movement is from the horizontal extended leg. Abduction and adduction are measured from the neutral position.

Rotation of the hip is assessed first with the thigh flexed to 90° and with the knee flexed. In osteoarthritis internal rotation is usually the first hip movement restricted. Rotation of the hip may also be assessed with the knee extended. Roll the hip with the knee straight.

Specific tests

With non-specific groin pain is it important to undertake a full clinical examination to exclude other significant injuries. In particular, it is essential to examine the inguinal canal when a sports hernia is suspected.

Groin pain

Groin pain is now almost fashionable. So many footballers have had groin surgery that all our patients know all about it. Patients are quite likely to ask to be referred directly for surgery and to have detailed knowledge about the anatomy and surgical technique. This is media medicine with the expectation that surgery can cure all groin pain.

Not all have a significant groin problem and not all those with groin pain require surgery. But groin pain is in the news and as general practitioners we ought to know about it. The media hype may cloud the most important feature of chronic groin pain: the serious effect that it can have on the performance of an athlete and how it destroys the sporting career of many amateur and professional footballers. There are a number of causes and the currently popular hernia repair is not the answer to them all. Adductor muscle sprain, adductor origin injury, osteitis pubis, stress fractures and inguinal hernia are just some of the other causes.

Sports hernia

The eponymous 'Gilmore's groin' describes a covert hernia. In most cases the diagnosis is made on symptoms and clinical signs alone. The patient has groin pain, usually on exertion. The signs are of groin tenderness on digital examination. It is occasionally possible to palpate a hernia if the athlete, usually a footballer, can increase abdominal pressure, by contracting the abdominal muscles. In most cases there is no obvious hernia, visible nor palpable, and tenderness is usually the only sign. The lesion causing the symptoms is usually a defect of the posterior wall of the inguinal canal. Investigations including herniography may not be definitive and surgery is often undertaken on clinical grounds alone. In most cases surgery does improve the symptoms but some surgeons remain sceptical. Because of the widespread knowledge about this problem and the popularity of surgery among footballers there is considerable pressure to refer, and on surgeons to operate. Return to sport takes about 6 weeks.

Adductor strain

Recurrent groin strain may be due to traction injuries of the adductor origin on the pubic bone. The pain is associated with resisted adduction, for example when kicking, and the pain is sudden and occurs on muscle contraction. The diagnosis may be made by demonstrating pain on resisted abduction. Adductor strains can become recurrent and then chronic so it is important to treat this injury appropriately. The player should rest until the acute pain has eased and then begin gradual rehabilitation. Muscle tears of the adductor muscle belly should be treated in the same manner as any acute muscle tear and they rarely cause chronic problems. After initial first aid treatment with a short period of rest, the injury is managed by progressive return to activity, stretching and strengthening. Other related acute muscle strain injury may occur at the lower fibres of the rectus abdominus.

Symphysitis pubis

This injury has a different symptom pattern with a nagging pain, worse during and after exercise. The injury is caused by increased stress across the symphysis usually in sports which require a sudden rotation. It can occur in ball sports especially with kicking but can also occur in field sports such as hockey which require sudden body movements and change of direction with a fixed resistant surface. When the rotation cannot be fully absorbed at the hips, the stress is transmitted across the pubic rami. With a severe injury there is movement at the symphysis although this is rarely felt by the athlete in spite of the excessive movement (2 mm) or instability seen on X-ray. The classic X-ray is the flamingo view which demonstrates movement of the symphysis when the patient stands on one leg. Increased bone activity may also be seen on a bone scan.

Osteitis pubis is an overuse injury that almost always gets better with rest, but rest is not usually welcomed by the athletes. Rather than advise complete rest one can redirect the training focus towards atraumatic activity such as cycling or swimming to maintain fitness. In this way the player can maintain aerobic fitness without the stress on the symphysis associated with running. If the injury is to a runner who is keen to maintain sport-specific fitness they can train in a pool wearing a flotation jacket, but it is impossible to mimic the activities of football. Hip flexibility may be an important factor in preventing osteitis pubis [2], so maintaining and increasing hip flexibility are an important components of rehabilitation. Supportive shorts have also been suggested as being of some benefit.

Stress fractures

Stress fractures of the pubic ramus can occur, particularly in distance runners. Interestingly, they are more common in women which may be because of the different anatomy and direction of stresses, although other factors may also be important. The treatment is rest.

Stress fractures of the neck of femur are of much more concern. The history is of the classic crescendo pain typical of the stress fracture, which increases in severity with time and eventually leads to night time bone pain. In female osteoporotic distant runners one must be especially vigilant and in the thin female distance runner, hip joint pain should be investigated thoroughly.

The angulation of the femoral neck means that there are two variants of the femoral stress fracture: a compression and distraction type. These occur on the upper and lower parts of the femoral neck respectively. Stress fractures of the upper cortex demand more urgent attention and the patient should be non-weight-bearing immediately as there is a serious risk of complete fracture, especially in older people.

Stress fractures of the lower part of the neck of the femur are more common in younger people. They also demand serious attention and the patient should be non-weight-bearing while symptomatic. They may need to use crutches for 4–6 weeks followed by a period of gradual graded rehabilitation. There is much less risk of complete fracture although a fracture that is not healing may occasionally require internal fixation. Femoral stress fractures require specialist attention and should always be referred to an orthopaedic surgeon.

Other causes of exercise-related hip pain include trochanteric bursitis, which occurs where the bursa over the greater trochanter of the femur becomes painful and inflamed. There is pain, usually on running, with local tenderness at the greater trochanter. The area over the bursa may feel soft and spongy. Topical anti-inflammatory agents may help, rest will ease the pain, but injection may be necessary. The trochanteric bursa lies over the greater trochanter. To inject the bursa, lie the patient on the unaffected side. The bursa is just superficial to the bone so advance the needle until the needle tip touches the bone and withdraw very slightly. It is sometimes possible to withdraw some fluid. Inject using 1–2 ml of local anaesthetic (lignocaine 1%) and short-acting steroid (10 mg hydrocortisone acetate).

Other important causes of hip pain

We must always consider the more common causes of hip pain in the young athlete including slipped femoral epiphysis and Perthes' disease. Irritable hip is a familiar diagnosis with associated synovitis, but this can occur also in the athlete. In the older patient osteoarthritis is common although this diagnosis is not always confined to the elderly and some younger ex-contact-sport players suffer from premature osteoarthritis. More rarely avascular necrosis of the neck of the femur occurs.

Athletes often ask about clicks in the groin. If this occurs over the greater trochanter this is usually due to the tensor fascia lata clicking as it crosses over the trochanteric bursa. It is more common in women because of their wider hips. If the click is on the front of the hip it may be due to the iliopsoas tendon as it clicks over a bony prominence. Iliopsoas bursitis also occurs but in most cases this is an ultrasound diagnosis and is treated by surgical excision of the bursa.

Injuries to the muscles of the thigh

Quadriceps

The quadriceps muscle group on the front of the thigh extends from its origin on the femur and ilium to its insertion first in the patella and then through the patella into the tibial tubercle (Figure 12.1). The rectus femoris has its origin on the anterior inferior iliac spine while the other three muscles, the vastus lateralis, vastus medialis and vastus intermedius, have their origin on the linea aspera and anterior femur. This muscle group is injured most often by contusion but it can also be torn. A muscle tear may be complete or partial. A partial muscle tear is treated using the principle of RICE as described earlier. Complete tears of the quadriceps occur most often in the muscle belly of the rectus femoris. There is a sudden tear with pain and muscle weakness. One can often palpate the defect on the front of thigh. This type of injury is

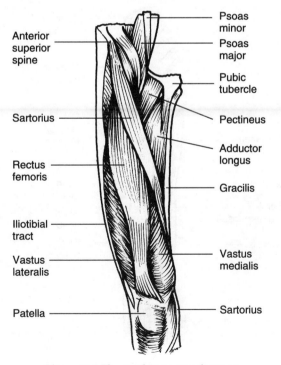

Figure 12.1 The quadriceps muscle group.

more common in older athletes and is usually associated with sudden unaccustomed exercise. It occurs typically with a sudden deceleration where there is a sudden contraction of the muscle as the player tries to stop. Surgical repair of this injury is almost impossible as the two ends of the muscle cannot be reattached. The initial treatment is the same as of any acute muscle tear and rehabilitation is focused on strengthening the remaining quadriceps muscle to compensate. Quadriceps muscle training, especially training of the vastus medialis obliquus is addressed below.

Hamstring

The hamstring muscles extend from the buttock to the knee (Figure 12.2). There are three separate muscles in this group: the semimembranosus, semitendinosus and biceps femoris. They all have their origin in the ischial tuberosity, although the

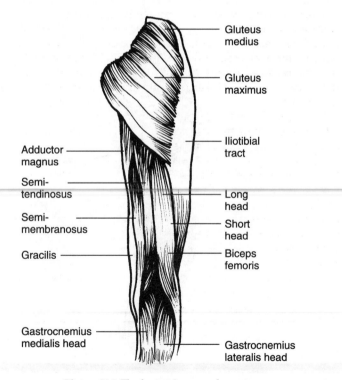

Figure 12.2 The hamstring muscle group.

biceps femoris has two heads and the short head has its origin on the posterolateral femur. The semimembranosus is inserted in the medial tibia and knee joint and the semitendinosus is inserted on the pes anserinus and then in the anteromedial tibia. These are on the medial side of the popliteal fossa. The biceps femoris is on the lateral side and is inserted into the proximal fibula.

Hamstring muscle tears and rehabilitation

Hamstring tears are common, especially in sprinting sports including the pure athletic sprint (such as 100 m and 200 m) and various types of football and field sports where sudden sprints and accelerations are an integral part of the game. The hamstrings are also vulnerable in jumping, hurdling and kicking sports. Hamstring tears occur in different parts of the muscle depending on the nature of the sport. Midmuscle tears are more common in sprinting, while tears at the origin occur most often in high hurdles. Recent work suggests that hamstring tears are more common when there is an imbalance between hamstrings and quadriceps muscle strength, so retraining and strengthening the hamstrings is an essential part of the rehabilitation after injury. As with all muscle injuries, hamstring tears are more common when the muscle is cold. A warm muscle is more plastic and less likely to rupture.

Knowing the aetiology of the injury and the type of sports in which such injuries occur we should be able to introduce an appropriate preventative programme. Prevention must include both warm-up and stretching. Stretching is important because a longer muscle is better able to absorb sudden forces and to avoid tear, while a shortened muscle is more prone to injury. A stretching programme is intended to extend the functional range of movement and any inequality in muscle length. A muscle previously injured has a tendency to shorten. Scar tissue contracts in healing so an injured muscle which has healed with some scaring is a shortened muscle. Fatigue may also be a factor. Hamstring injuries can occur early in a game with a sudden contraction in a cold muscle, but also occur towards the end of a game when fatigue means that the muscles may be less well coordinated and may be more likely to tear.

The symptoms associated with a hamstring tear depend on the severity of the injury. With mild or first degree tears an athlete may not be aware of any problem until after the game or training session. The first symptoms may be a nagging ache with minimal signs, full range of movement and no pain on exertion or stretching. With a more severe, second or third degree tear, the athlete is aware when the injury occurs and feels a sudden rip or pop as the muscle tears. There is pain and perhaps a palpable gap in the muscle. This gap may be palpable immediately but soon fills due to bleeding and swelling. Bruising is not usually seen at the site of the injury at first but will track downwards and may only be seen a few days after the injury when there is discoloration at the back of the knee. This is disconcerting for the patient who wonders why there is bruising at the knee not realising that this is due to distal tracking. With a severe tear there is marked swelling and pain and the athlete will be unable to put his/her foot to the ground.

Mild to moderate hamstring tears are most common and should be treated actively. The initial treatment is usefully described using the acronym RICE. Rest means rest from any athletic sports for at least 24 hours. Ice helps reduce swelling and blood loss. A thigh compression bandage helps in two ways. It provides some compression force helping to reduce swelling but also serves as a useful reminder of their injury and that they should be resting. Physiotherapy has a role in the early stages where ultrasound may help reduce the blood clot and oedema. Early mobilisation is the rule with walking as soon as the initial pain and swelling have eased. At about 48 hours the athlete can begin gentle stretching but within the limits of pain. Pain indicates that the tissues are being stressed excessively and is a signal to stop. The next stage is rehabilitation. Return to sport is only allowed when the athlete can do all the movements associated with that sport. Rehabilitation will begin with gentle jogging gradually increasing the intensity, but still within the limits of pain and if there is any sensation of pulling or tension they should stop immediately. Ideally the athletes will have ultrasound and some gentle active and passive stretching immediately after training. Rehabilitation should also include some strengthening exercises for the hamstrings. One week after the injury the athlete should be able to sprint in training, but should still have regular ultrasound and be doing active and passive stretching before and after exercise. Non-steroidal anti-inflammatory drugs may also be of benefit. When the athlete can do all the movements associated with the game in a non-competitive environment they may then progress to participation in the sport. Hamstring strengthening exercises should also form part of the long-term rehabilitation. With a severe muscle tear, all these stages of treatment are more protracted. The first stage is much prolonged as there is considerable pain and swelling and the patient cannot walk with comfort. Strengthening exercise can begin when the athlete has recovered the full pain-free range of movement. An introductory programme would include some hamstring curls, and there are weight benches in most gymnasia designed especially for this exercise. It is best, however, to get some expert advice from a specialised trainer.

Management of hamstring injury

The acronym TREAT reminds us of the components of injury management.

T*reatment*
Treatment begins with rest, ice, compression and elevation. There is initial immobilisation with encouragement of activity to achieve a full pain-free range of movement. The physiotherapy includes ultrasound, and non-steroidal anti-inflammatory medication may be used.

R*ehabilitation*
Begins with gentle stretching, muscle exercise is then resumed with isometric strengthening initially and later isotonic and isokinetic submaximal muscle contractions. Physiotherapy will include heat, massage and electrical treatments.

E*xercise*
Later exercise includes progressive dynamic exercises, jogging, running, swimming, cycling, strengthening exercises and stretching exercises.

A*ctivity*
When able to return to full activity the athlete can try full sprinting, jumping and return to all the non-competitive activities of the sport.

T*arget*
The target is the return to competition. It is essential that the return to sport also includes efforts to prevent recurrence of the injury. This means a preparticipation prevention programme with warm-up, stretching and protective heat retaining clothes. Warmdown should include strengthening agonists and antagonists.

Chronic hamstring injuries

A chronic hamstring injury is simply a recurrent injury which has not been fully rehabilitated. Re-injury and recurrent injury are common where the athlete returns to sport before all the stages of rehabilitation have completed.

Hamstring tendinitis causes an aching pain along the tendon and is due to overuse. There may be some swelling and tenderness of the tendon. It should be treated with rest, ice and anti-inflammatory medication either as tablets or gel. It is a common cycling injury and occurs if there are abnormal leg movements when pedalling, for example if the cyclist rotates the leg during the pedal stroke.

References

1 Andersen KV, Bovim G. Impotence and nerve entrapment in long distance amateur cyclist. *Acta Neurol Scand* 1997; **95**: 233–40.
2 Fricker PA. Management of groin pain in athletes. *Br J Sports Med* 1997; **31**: 97–101.

13 Injuries of the lower leg

Knee examination

Orthopaedic texts will give a full description of the correct technique in examination of the knee. This checklist is to act as a reminder and gives some indication of what the underlying problem may be. It is of course a very basic guide and cannot possibly be comprehensive. If in doubt a specialist opinion should be sought.

Knee examination checklist

Inspection standing	• weight bearing • walking • swelling • Q angle
Inspection supine	• muscle wasting • effusion
Palpation	• apprehension test • test for effusion • Clarke's sign
Movements	• active • passive
Ligaments	• collaterals
Anterior drawer test	
Lachman's test	
Pivot shift	
Meniscus/McMurray/Apley test	

Inspection

Look for swelling, effusion, muscle wasting and the position of the patella. Knee swelling is usually due to an effusion but may be due to a haemarthrosis. The history is probably the best indication of the cause; a haemarthrosis occurs immediately after an injury and usually indicates a more serious injury either to the menisci or the cruciate ligament while an effusion may occur as a result of a more chronic inflammation. The first indication of an effusion is loss of contour and filling of the dimples at the side of the knee. One may detect a small effusion by milking fluid down into the joint and seeing the subtle change in contour in these dimples. Many textbooks describe the tibial tap which occurs in a moderate effusion. This is the sensation that one can feel when pushing the patella down to knock against the femur. The tibial tap may be present with a moderate effusion but with a large effusion or haemarthrosis the joint is usually too tense to allow enough patella movement. Muscle wasting may be obvious but usually only if there is a large loss of muscle bulk. More subtle wasting occurs in the vastus medialis and this occurs early in any knee injury and is non-specific.

Retraining of the vastus medialis is a central part of the rehabilitation after any knee injury. Severe muscle wasting can be seen even with the muscles relaxed, but it is usually more obvious when the muscle is tensed and can be objectively assessed by measurement using a tape measure.

The position of the patella may indicate an increased likelihood of anterior knee pain or dislocation. Other problems that may be seen on inspection include bursitis, either due to housemaid's or clergyman's knee, inflammation of the fat pad, or the swollen prominent tibial tubercle of Osgood–Schlatter disease. The knee should be inspected both standing and lying.

Active movements

Observing the patient walking, one may see a limp, abnormal movement or muscle imbalance. One can also estimate the 'Q' angle, which is the angle between a line connecting the anterior superior iliac spine and the midpoint of the patella, with the vertical. Look then at active flexion and extension with the patient lying down to see if there are full and equal ranges of movement. Limitation of the range of either parameter may indicate a mechanical block, perhaps by a loose body or a displaced meniscus, or limitation because of the discomfort of an effusion or soft tissue problem due to pain within the muscle or tendon.

Passive movements of flexion or extension may help confirm the range of movement and help indicate the cause of the problem.

Resisted movements

Resisted flexion and extension will give an indication of muscle strength. Neurological problems can be detected, although these are not usually a feature of sports injuries.

Palpation

An effusion may be confirmed by palpation and even a mild effusion can be milked down into the joint and seen as a moving dimple. Almost two thirds of the reverse side of the patella can be palpated and tenderness may point to the cause of anterior knee pain. The joint line should be palpated as tenderness along the joint line suggests meniscus injury. In contrast, injured collateral ligaments may not be tender at the joint line as the collateral ligaments, the medial ligament in particular, extend quite distant from the joint line.

Collateral ligaments

The medial and lateral collateral ligaments provide the lateral stability of the knee and are often injured in contact sport. It is essential in testing the collateral ligaments that the thigh muscles are relaxed. A method of relaxing these muscles is to take the weight of the leg by lifting the leg and fixing it by tucking it under the examiner's arm. There will always be some lateral movement (<5°) in the knee joint but there should be a pain-free endpoint to this joint movement. Collateral ligament injuries are graded according to the severity of the injury but are almost always managed conservatively.

Cruciate ligaments

These ligaments criss-cross the knee joint internally and provide the forward–backward stability of the knee. To provide this anterior–posterior stability the ligaments must be internal and oblique. Their purpose is to prevent forward and backward slippage of the tibia on the femur. They take their name from their position on the tibia so that the anterior cruciate goes from the anterior of the articular surface of the tibia and is attached at the posterior articular surface of the femur. Its purpose is to prevent the tibia from moving forwards so its integrity is tested by attempting to pull the tibia forwards – the anterior drawer test. The posterior cruciate prevents backward movement and while there is no single specific test, complete tears will allow the tibia to sag backwards from its neutral position. Because tight or tense hamstrings can stop the tibia moving forwards in the anterior drawer test, it may be more useful to use Lachman's test. This is simply the anterior drawer test performed at 15° of flexion. Diagnosis of anterior cruciate ligament injury is difficult and is often missed [1]. It is important for the sports physician to become expert in the anterior cruciate assessment (Figure 13.1).

There is a more specialist functional test of the anterior cruciate ligament. The anterior cruciate, while it prevents forward and backward movement when the knee is flexed, also has a key role in keeping the knee stable when players are changing direction, such as in cutting and side stepping. If the anterior cruciate is torn, players feel insecure when changing direction and often describe how their knee feels unstable. Their knee may indeed give way when they try to change direction. The pivot shift test is a functional test which stresses the knee in this same anterolateral direction. Written descriptions of this test sound very complicated and it is most easily understood in the context of the natural movement that occurs in sport. It attempts to reproduce the movements that occur when a patient tries to suddenly change direction or cut. Thus the test measures anterolateral instability.

To do the pivot shift test, begin with the leg in full extension and apply a valgus stress with internal tibial rotation while flexing the knee. This may cause subluxation of the tibia relative to the femur with a palpable (often painful) clunk. Rather than try to understand the test from text, it is much easier to learn how to do it from a demonstration. There are other functional tests of instability of both the anterior and posterior cruciate ligaments but these are most easily learned when the basics are mastered.

The posterior cruciate ligament protects the knee from abnormal posterior movements. Clearly this laxity will be seen on the anterior drawer sign also, but the key to detecting if it is the posterior cruciate ligament that is deficient is the starting point. If, with the knee flexed to 90°, the tibia has slipped posterior then the posterior cruciate ligament is lax or ruptured.

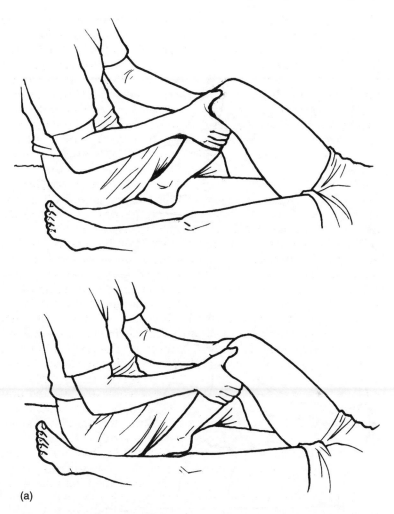

(a)

Figure 13.1 Diagnosis of anterior cruciate ligament injury. (a) The anterior drawer test. (b) Lachman's test of anterior stability: leg held in hand or leg held between arm and body of physician.

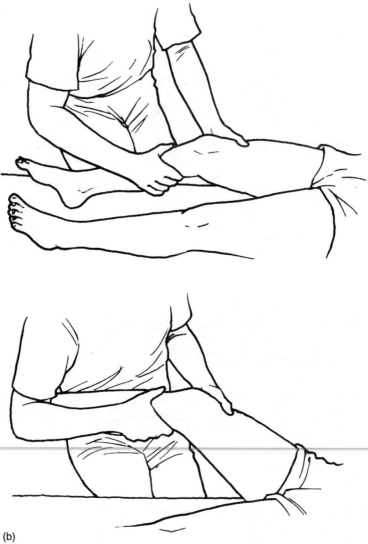

(b)

Meniscus tests

McMurray and Apley described tests of meniscus injury. Before arthroscopy was commonplace and MRI scans became readily available, these tests were popular. Meniscus injury is usually suspected from the history and the suspicion heightened by joint line tenderness and even a palpable joint line bulge on knee flexion. Arthroscopy and MRI have cast doubt on the accuracy of McMurray's and Apley's tests and they are now almost obsolete.

Knee joint injuries

A description of the site of the pain and how it occurred can give some indication of the aetiology. The anterior cruciate ligament usually tears in a twisting movement, or with twisting and varus/valgus or hyperextension. It may occur together with an injury to the lateral or medial meniscus or with a collateral ligament.

The meniscus injury occurs classically when there is a twisting movement on a weight bearing fixed foot. This explains how it can occur in a tackle in football where there is a forced twisting movement with the foot is planted in the ground. In those over 40 years of age the meniscus may already have undergone some degeneration, and a meniscus injury may occur following relatively minor trauma, even after a simple movement such as squatting. In those who present with symptoms suggestive of a meniscus injury there are two options. In some cases the symptoms may settle with conservative management but persistent symptoms may indicate the need for surgery. If the patient is symptomatic and the MRI demonstrates a meniscus problem the treatment of choice is arthroscopic surgery.

With chronic knee pain, a patient may indicate vaguely over the knee cap. This suggests patellofemoral pain. If they point to the joint line, either medially or laterally this may suggest a meniscus injury. Locking or giving way, while the classic description of meniscus injury, may not always be predictive. The patient's understanding of the term 'locking' may differ from the clinician's understanding. True locking, when there is a springy block to extension indicates obstruction to the extensor mechanism which may be due to a meniscus or foreign body. Pseudo locking occurs where the patient feels unable to extend the knee because of generalised pain, especially anterior knee pain. 'Giving way' is another typical presentation of a knee problem. A knee may give way due to reflex muscle relaxation or ligamentous instability. Reflex muscle relaxation may occur due to severe pain but can occur with an anterior cruciate ligament injury, especially when cutting or changing direction, because the ACL is the key anterolateral knee stabiliser.

Simple anterior and lateral X-rays may not always give a good indication of injury. For investigation of anterior knee pain it may be necessary to ask for skyline views to view the posterior patella.

Management and rehabilitation from an anterior cruciate ligament injury

The anterior cruciate ligament prevents anterior movement of the tibia. The anterior cruciate ligament has its origin on the tibial spine and tracks backwards through intercondylar notch to insertion on the femur. Rupture of the anterior cruciate allows the forward movement of the tibia that is tested using the anterior drawer test and Lachman's test described above. More important, however, is the anterolateral instability which will greatly limit the ability to play sport.

Immediately after an injury, it may be possible to detect ligament instability, but after the haemarthrosis develops further ligament assessment is impossible. A haemarthrosis should be drained in the aseptic environment of a theatre. When the knee settles down, there is time to assess joint stability and to decide on long-term management. Many elite level professional athletes have an almost immediate surgical repair but the alternative, for the majority of the sporting population, is to consider surgery only after failure of conservative management. Surgical repair, if undertaken, is only the first step and functional rehabilitation with full recovery and return to sport requires a long-term commitment. It may be 9–12 months after surgery before the athlete can return to the previous level of sport, although occasionally rehabilitation may be quicker.

The decision on progression to surgery is undertaken by the athlete and surgeon together. The key factors are the importance of sport to the patient, and the type of sport. The ability to cut or change direction quickly is the functional measure of anterolateral instability. If a young high level sports performer wishes to return to top level sport and is prepared to make the commitment to the rehabilitation programme then surgery is appropriate. Many older, less serious players will be happy to undertake a period of rehabilitation and tolerate instability. Those who have had a cruciate injury with or without reconstruction are at increased risk of long-term osteoarthritis so the decision on surgery should be made on the basis of intention to return to sport.

Surgical reconstruction of the anterior cruciate ligament has evolved but it is still not perfect and is complicated by the difficulty in achieving both an anatomical and functional repair. Initial attempts to use carbon fibre or Dacron were relatively unsuccessful and at present surgeons generally use autografts taken either from the patellar tendon or hamstring tendon. Surgeons now encourage early mobilisation and rehabilitation. Early mobilisation is the key to management after surgery but the key to successful rehabilitation is perhaps not so much rehabilitation after surgery, as muscle training and preparation before surgery. If the knee is functionally limited, there may already be considerable muscle atrophy. Prehospital preparation aims to train and maintain the muscle function. Rehabilitation after surgery is just as important, if not more so, than the surgery itself. Each surgeon has his or her own treatment and rehabilitation protocol but the general principles are the same. The outcomes from different techniques do not appear to be that different [2].

The early phase

Surgeons often use a brace after operation to prevent full extension, but encourage movement within the limitations allowed by the brace. Continuous passive movement (CPM) is usually an integral part of early management. As the knee settles down the range of movement and intensity of activity is increased. In the first 2 weeks the patient will increase the intensity and range of exercise through resistance exercises and mobilisation.

The middle phase

Physiotherapy increases the strength and range of movement aiming for full range of movement and muscle strength at 6 weeks. Most of the rehabilitation exercises during this phase are non-weight-bearing.

The late phase

From 6 weeks to 6 months the patient continues functional rehabilitation. Beginning with low intensity running and introducing sharp turns and cutting movements no sooner than 12 weeks. Return to top level sport is unlikely before 6–9 months and this usually means that a player loses a complete year as the athlete can rarely return within the season. This has an advantage, however, in that it usually enforces a prolonged late phase of rehabilitation. A player, regardless of the game, should only be allowed to return to competitive sport when they can undertake full sport-specific activities and muscle strength is within 10% of its previous level.

Conservative treatment

Many knees can function very well without surgery providing they are retrained appropriately. For those not wishing to return to top level sport, a strengthening and rehabilitation programme may allow the return of the patient to a satisfactory activity level. Such rehabilitation includes training both the agonists and antagonists with the quadriceps and hamstrings equally important. To prevent anterior movement of the tibia, as occurs in an anterior cruciate deficient knee, hamstring muscle tone and strength may be considered more critical. Sport-specific rehabilitation can begin at about 3 months.

Treatment

Rest, ice, compression and elevation are used. There is initial immobilisation with later encouragement of activity to achieve pain-free range of movement. Physiotherapy includes ultrasound and non-steroidal anti-inflammatory medication is used.

Rehabilitation

Gentle stretching is used to resume muscle exercise, with isometric strengthening initially and later isotonic and isokinetic submaximal muscle contractions. Physiotherapy includes heat, massage and electrical treatments.

Exercise

The next stage introduces progressive dynamic exercises: jogging, running, swimming and cycling. Strengthening exercises and stretching exercises are important.

Activity
Later there is full sprinting, jumping and return to all the non-competitive activities of the sport.

Target
The target is return to competition in sport. It is essential that the return to sport also includes efforts to prevent recurrence of the injury. This means a pre-participation prevention programme with warm-up, stretching and protective heat retaining clothes. The warm-down period should be used for strengthening agonists and antagonists.

Anterior knee pain

Anterior knee pain is one of the most common presentations in primary care. To help doctors advise patients with this condition, here is a leaflet which may be copied and given to patients in the consulting room.

Patient management of anterior knee pain

Anterior knee pain is one of the most common injuries in sport, and known by athletes as runner's knee, rower's knee or cyclist's knee. That it has these names shows how common it is in these sports. You may feel the pain behind the knee cap or sometimes just at the inner edge. The pain is due to abnormal movement of the knee cap. The smooth movement of the knee cap depends on equal muscle pull on both sides of the knee cap. This smooth action can be altered because the knee cap is pulled out of position or because there is too much load.

Excess load

The quadriceps muscle straightens the leg by pulling on the lower leg across the kneecap which acts as a pulley. With too much load the knee cap is forced against the femur. This can happen in cycling or in weight training. Healthy muscle can exert a force of 42 pounds per square inch and the quadriceps is a most powerful muscle exerting a force up to 700 pounds. In cycling, for example, the key to prevention is cadence because if the cyclist pedals at a higher rate using a lower gear there is less load with each pedal stroke. In weight training the athlete should not squat so deep.

Abnormal tracking

If the quadriceps muscle tends to pull the knee cap out of position, this will cause friction on the back of the knee cap. Prevention and treatment of this knee pain means ensuring that the muscles act in a balanced way.

Muscle balance

There are four muscle groups in the quadriceps, but only one of these muscle groups pulls the knee cap inwards. Any imbalance in the quadriceps muscle pulling on the kneecap tends to pull the knee cap out of its natural groove. The muscle on the inside is called the vastus medialis and it is perhaps the most important of the quadriceps muscle group. A part of this muscle known as vastus medialis obliquus (VMO) is particularly important and it is on the inner side just above the knee.

You can see your own VMO by tensing the thigh muscle and the VMO bulges just above the knee on the inside. This particular muscle is unfortunately very prone to weakening or wasting and when this happens the kneecap is drawn out of its natural position. Even a minor knee injury may lead to some wasting of the VMO which occurs very early in any knee injury. Retraining of the

▶

quadriceps, and the VMO in particular, is an essential part of rehabilitation from any knee injury, however minor.

Quadriceps muscle training

Training the VMO requires specific exercises which take into consideration the particular features of the muscle. The VMO is most active in the last 15° of extension, the final part of leg straightening, so standard weight training exercises such as squats and leg extension exercises are of little use and more specialised training exercises are necessary.

These exercises may be static or dynamic. The static exercises are often called 'quads drill' and go as follows. With the leg straight, tighten the muscles to draw the kneecap upwards and towards you and try to pull as hard as possible using the muscles on the front of the thigh. Follow the rule of tens: hold the contraction for 10 seconds, relax for 10 seconds and do this 10 times. This exercise is often taught to patients after knee surgery.

Dynamic exercises are those which involve movement or shortening of the muscle, for example when lifting weights. Even in dynamic exercise the muscle contraction should be within no more than 15° of flexion from full extension in order to train the VMO.

A typical exercise is as follows. Hold the leg over the end of a weight bench in 15° of flexion and straighten the leg. This will ensure the use of VMO. To increase the load and train the VMO more effectively, add light weights of no more than 2 pounds initially. This exercise may be easily done at home over the end of the bed. To add extra resistance once could, for example, hook a carrier bag over the foot and add weights such as books etc.

The 'squeeze pillow' exercise is combination of static and dynamic exercise. With the leg horizontal, place a pillow under the slightly flexed knee. The pillow is squeezed as hard as possible with the back of the leg. In this exercise the VMO is contracted with the leg in partial flexion and with a pillow under a slightly bent leg.

With anterior knee pain the patient should try to stay off their knees as much as possible. If you are a plumber or electrician (or clergyman!) this may be difficult, otherwise leave the gardening or carpet laying to someone else.

Sometimes your doctor will prescribe anti-inflammatory medication. While this may help reduce the inflammation at the back of the kneecap, it treats only the symptoms and not the cause of the problem. Try to think of the cause of the problem. Anti-inflammatory tablets may sometimes have side-effects and in particular can cause stomach upset. If you have an ulcer they are best avoided. Happily these anti-inflammatories are now available as a gel or foam which helps avoid some of the side-effects of the tablets.

Corticosteroid injections may reduce inflammation in the joint temporarily but they always cause some breakdown of tissue within the joint. Injection into the joint may offer a short-term answer, but

▶

only stores up greater problems for the future. Injections into the knee joint are not recommended, except in the elderly.

There are many operations described in the treatment of anterior knee pain so you can be sure that no one treatment really works well! Try to avoid surgery as the time spent in surgery, recovery, and rehabilitation may be longer than you would spend if you simply let the inflammation ease by rest.

Knee pain is the curse of the athlete, especially the rower and cyclist, and must be treated seriously. Part of the macho image of sport is the ability to suffer! Knee pain is not a pain to be suffered, it will only get worse. Treat it seriously and with respect!

Anterior knee pain of this sort used to be diagnosed as chondromalacia patella, but it is known from arthroscopic findings that this term is not anatomically correct. Measures to smooth or shave the cartilage are not always effective.

The pain is an ache, felt as a general knee pain, and patients often cannot point to any specific location but indicate vaguely towards the top of the patella. Pain below the patella in adolescents may be due to Osgood–Schlatter disease.

Anterior knee pain may be reproduced by compression on the patella during quadriceps tension as in Clarke's sign (but this is a rather non-specific sign). The pain is usually worse after a period of inactivity, for example on getting up to walk after sitting for a while, a symptom described as the 'cinema sign'. The pain is often worse when driving, and patients typically mention pain on descending stairs or walking down hill. It is unusual for these patients to describe pain on ascending stairs.

Orthotics

It may occur that patella maltracking is due to foot problems such as hyperpronation which can be treated by prescription of orthotics by a sport physiotherapist or podiatrist.

Medial plica

Runners and cyclists may describe a pain on the medial joint line, associated with a click. This is a form of anterior knee pain where there is inflammation of a fold of synovium anteromedially. There may be tenderness on palpation. This is medial plica syndrome.

Iliotibial band friction syndrome

This is a common and rewarding condition to treat in general practice. The iliotibial band crosses the lateral femoral condyle at the knee and the iliotibial band can flick back and forward across the condyle causing a friction-type irritation, especially in distance running. The athlete will complain of pain and is tender over the lateral femoral condyle. The Noble compression test describes tenderness over the lateral condyle on extension of the knee while putting pressure on the condyle. Treatment is directed at stretching the iliotibial band so that it causes less friction, and by injection of corticosteroid which reduces inflammation.

Bursitis

Most general practitioners are familiar with the common presentations of bursitis that occur around the knee (housemaid's knee and clergyman's knee). A similar bursitis occurs at the elbow. These are the most common but there are many bursae present in the body which can become similarly swollen and tender. In sport this may be due to the nature of the sport and are most often associated with overuse. Those most common are the pes anserinus bursa and the trochanteric bursa. Generally they are associated with friction-type injuries or overuse. Like all bursae they may be treated by drainage and injection of a small quantity of a short-acting steroid such as hydrocortisone acetate, but they often recur.

Osgood–Schlatter disease

This is an apophysitis which occurs in adolescents and presents as pain and swelling at the upper part of the tibia, just where the quadriceps tendon is attached to the bone. Osgood–Schlatter disease is a traction injury and the pain is due to inflammation of the insertion of the tendon into the tibia. It is a very common injury and occurs at a time when the young athlete is most keen and enthusiastic. At this age, the muscle and tendon are often stronger than the bone, so with frequent and sustained contraction of the muscle, the tendon pulls hard on the bony attachment causing this traction injury and pain. Patients complain of a chronic ache and pain on ascending stairs. The pain is made worse by sport and there is often a tender swelling just below the knee. Typically the young sportsperson, almost always a boy, is upset that they cannot play sport, often football, because of the pain. They are usually very keen, often talented players who may be playing every day or even more than once each day. Their parents may be equally upset.

The only appropriate treatment is to reduce the stress on the tendon attachment which, in effect, means rest from sport. This is frustrating because they probably sustained the injury principally because they were so keen and enthusiastic in the first place. There is, however, no substitute for rest, but only from the sport that caused the problem. To maintain cardiovascular fitness the young athlete can still swim. Realistically it is difficult for young athletes to rest and most practitioners let the young person choose their own level of activity. Rupture is extremely rare and pain is usually the worst symptom.

Other less common knee problems

These include osteochondritis dessicans, where a small piece of cartilage becomes dislodged from the medial femoral condyle and is present as a loose body within the joint. It commonly occurs in teenagers where the presenting symptoms are of locking, giving way, effusion or pain. Surgery may be required either to remove a small loose body or to replace a larger fragment. A meniscal cyst may occur at the joint line. This is usually associated with a meniscus tear and is managed surgically.

A Baker's cyst occurs in the popliteal fossa. In most cases this is left alone as it causes few symptoms, does no harm and often resolves on its own. Occasionally a Baker's cyst may rupture causing pain and swelling in the calf which can be confused with a DVT. Other bursae may occur at the front of the knee: prepatella and infrapatella bursitis. Pes anserinus bursitis may occur on the medial side just proximal to the insertion of the pes anserinus.

Shin splints

The patient may tell you that they have shin splints. They are describing a clinical syndrome rather than a specific diagnosis as shin splints is a generic term used by lay people to describe exercise-related shin pain. The term includes all the common causes of shin pain including stress fractures, compartment syndromes and periostitis.

Stress fractures

The history of pain associated with a stress fracture or fatigue fracture is classic and described as crescendo type pain. It is an exercise-related pain which increases in severity with the duration of exercise. As it becomes worse, the pain begins earlier and earlier after starting exercise so that eventually pain begins as soon as the exercise begins. Later there may be night pain. Such injuries usually occur in weight-bearing activities and the most common sites are in the lower leg associated with running. Stress fractures can also occur in the upper limb and the ribs. They can occur in spine as spondylolysis.

A stress fracture or fatigue fracture is an overuse injury where microfractures occur associated with repetitive stress. The natural shock absorbancy of the body is unable to cope with this sustained impact. If there is a biomechanical abnormality then there can be additional stresses. The injured bone does not have an opportunity to recover and eventually what was a microfracture becomes an obvious fracture. On examination there may be some local swelling and tenderness, especially on tapping the bone over the fracture site. In the early stages there are no X-ray changes but with continued repetitive stress callus forms as the bone attempts to repair and this may be visible on plain X-ray. Eventually a fracture line is seen. Stress fractures, while undetectable by plain X-ray in the early stages, may be seen as a hot spot on a bone scan. CT scan and MRI are also useful in further investigation. The treatment is rest, but like most overuse injuries, the rest is directed only at the injured part and means rest from the causative activity. The most common sites for stress fractures are the lower $\frac{1}{3}$ tibia where almost 50% of stress fractures occur, and the fibula, neck of femur and metatarsal where they occur usually due to running or dancing. The athlete can maintain fitness through swimming or cycling and should rest, usually for about 4 weeks.

Prevention is possible. Stress fractures occur due to recurrent microtrauma from the same repetitive movement and impact, so our aim in prevention is to modify training in order to reduce the repetitive trauma, while still maintaining some training stimulus. Prevention is a balance between sport-specific training and the risk of overuse injury.

Tibial stress fractures associated with running are avoided by reducing foot impact and resultant bone stress. This can be achieved at three levels. First, the athlete can change their running surface. Impact stress and related injuries can be reduced by training on a more forgiving surface, such as grass, or alternating the surfaces used. Impact can be reduced by changing one's shoe and using shoes with a more effective shock absorbing mid-sole. There are many such shoes available. Impact stress can also be related to intrinsic factors to do with the athlete themselves. If they are overweight or have a running style or biomechanical abnormality that increases the impact at foot strike, stress-related injury is more likely. Some of these factors can be modified so that weight loss can reduce foot strike impact and some biomechanical abnormalities can be modified by shoes or orthotics, but some people were not made to run and will always have a high impact running technique. Stress fractures can also occur because of the nature of a running programme which includes high mileage in the early stages when bones are unaccustomed to the stress of running, It may be necessary to stop the programme and begin again increasing the intensity and duration more slowly. In most cases a stress fracture is diagnosed on history alone, the investigation may be carried out if there is open access to radiology but the management can be entirely in general practice.

The first stage of treatment is to alter the type of training and use other forms of exercise that include endurance fitness but do not have repetitive impact. Suitable sports would be cycling, swimming or rowing. Any biomechanical abnormality should be corrected using orthotic or appropriately modified footwear. Rest from the activity that caused the injury is essential. The runner must stop running and dancer stop dancing, but additional training may add to the problem. So the runner or dancer should avoid other similar activities such as step aerobics. The duration of rest depends on the severity of the injury, but is likely to be more than 4 weeks.

Treatment of stress fractures

Treatment
Rest is the only appropriate immediate treatment. Non-steroidal anti-inflammatory medication can help reduce pain but should not be used to enable the patient to continue the activity. Other treatments have little effect and physiotherapy, particularly ultrasound, could make the problem worse.

Rehabilitation
While resting the injured leg the athlete will be keen to maintain cardiovascular fitness. One can continue a running programme in a pool using a flotation jacket. Alternatively the athlete may wish to cycle or row. Sprinting, intervals and endurance work can all be undertaken on a bike. A biomechanical assessment should be undertaken during this period, and factors which could have increased impact, hyperpronation for example, should be identified and the appropriate orthotics supplied.

E*xercise*
When the pain has gone, the athlete may consider return to sport-specific training. Initially this should be very gradual, alternating weight-bearing and non-weight-bearing activity. To reduce the impact stress they should run only on soft surfaces (which usually means grass). They should wear well cushioned running shoes and orthotics if indicated by the biomechanical assessment.

A*ctivity*
At first, the main fitness programme should be undertaken without weight-bearing and running only introduced very gradually. With time more sport-specific training can be undertaken. But, if there is any exercise related pain, the athlete must stop immediately.

T*arget*
The target is the return to competitive sport. It is essential to include a preventive strategy to avoid recurrence of the injury. This means running on an appropriate surface, varying the training to avoid overuse, proper shoes, alternating shoes and surfaces and orthotics if indicated.

Compartment syndromes

Compartment syndromes occur where there is compression of muscle within one of the muscle compartments of the lower leg. An acute compartment syndrome, usually as a result of trauma, should present to an accident and emergency department, so for practical purposes the general practitioner need only be concerned about the chronic compartment syndrome. There are four main compartments in the lower leg, three of which are surrounded by a firm fibrous capsule. The anterior compartment which contains the tibialis anterior, extensor digitorum longus and extensor hallucis longus muscles is the compartment most frequently affected. The deep posterior compartment which includes tibialis posterior, flexor digitorum longus and flexor hallucis longus is also sometimes a problem. The lateral compartment contains the peroneal muscles: superficial and longus. The superficial posterior compartment does not suffer compartment syndrome as it is loosely enveloped.

These calf muscles hypertrophy with training and, because the compartment is closed, this may raise intercompartmental pressure. Diagnosis is based on the history which describes an exercise related pain, somewhat similar to the pain of a stress fracture, but the pain is more vague and not localised to bone. The diagnosis is made on pressure studies, but these can only be undertaken at specialised centres. Rest will always temporarily reduce the symptoms and prolonged rest will lead to reduction in muscle size with reduced pressure. Training will of course lead to hypertrophy and recurrence of symptoms. Excessive muscle hypertrophy may be as a result of a biomechanical abnormality. If there is suspicion of a compartment syndrome the patient should be referred to hospital for investigation and perhaps surgery. There is no place for orthotics before investigation as these may simply add to the pressures. Medial tibial stress syndrome is due to periostitis which causes pain along the bone edge and occurs because of traction on the bone edge. It occurs with muscle activity and is diagnosed on history and ultimately on bone scan.

Examination of the foot and ankle

Inspection

Examine the athlete standing first and look from all directions at the ankle joint and the Achilles' tendon. Inspection may reveal swelling, bruising and anatomical abnormalities. Rather than list every possible anatomical problem, the key areas to examine are the Achilles' tendon to look for abnormalities, the ankle joint for swelling, and feet and toe abnormalities. Look for swelling, effusion, asymmetry and bruising. An ankle effusion is unusual and not always obvious. External swelling at the site of ligament sprains is much more common. An effusion may be due to a more chronic inflammation. Bursitis may occur either superficial or deep to the Achilles' tendon. The Achilles' tendon is usually obvious. The ankle should be inspected both standing and non-weight-bearing.

Palpation

Palpate around the ankle joint and include the foot. Palpation of the foot and ankle should include all the bony landmarks and tendon insertions. Problems occur commonly at the base of the 5th metatarsal, and at the navicular. Footballer's ankle may cause pain on the anterior tibia at the ankle joint. Look, in particular, for pain and tenderness at the malleoli and along the ligaments.

Palpate the fibula, at the lateral malleolus and proximal to the tibiofibular joint. Palpate along the tendons to their insertion and in particular palpate the 5th metatarsal and the navicular. Palpate also the sinus tarsi.

The Achilles' tendon may be palpated along its length from its calcaneal insertion to the musculotendonous junction. Diffuse swelling may indicate inflammation and palpable nodules may indicate degeneration. The tendon will be tender if inflammed. If there is any doubt about it being intact Simmond's or Thompson's test will confirm.

Active movements

Observe the ankle with the patient walking. Walking is the essential functional test. Also observe ankle flexion and extension from the front and from the rear, looking in particular at the Achilles' tendon. There may be a limp or abnormal movement. Ask the patient to go onto tip toes. Then ask the patient to squat and observe the direction of the Achilles' tendon. Some clinicians believe that the direction of the Achilles' in a half squat is the best indication of hyperpronation. Examine active flexion and extension with the patient lying down to see if there are full and equal ranges of movement. Passive movements of flexion or extension may help confirm the range of movement and help indicate the cause of the problem.

Resisted movements

Resisted flexion and extension will give an indication of muscle strength. Palpate also the peroneal tendons for slippage.

Passive movements

These should include flexion and extension and forefoot movements.

Collateral ligaments

The ankle is anatomically quite stable, but is most vulnerable to inversion injury. The medial collateral ligament is a fan shaped ligament while the lateral ligaments include three main components. The antero and posterior talofibular are from the neck and body of talus respectively, and the calcaneo fibular ligament.

Functional tests

These include an observation of the Achilles' tendon on knee flexion. The angle of the Achilles' tendon in mid-flexion may indicate a hyperpronation abnormality. Podiatrists and bio-mechanists describe the position of the Achilles' tendon with the foot in the neutral position but detecting the neutral position is subjective and may be unreliable. The anterior drawer sign tests the anterior talofibular ligament and excessive movement may indicate instability.

Special tests

Examine the ankle joint including the drawer sign. This is similar to the drawer sign at the knee. Hold the heel in the cup of the hand and try to draw the ankle forward holding the distal tibia and fibula with the other hand. Examine internal and external rotation. The syndesmosis is examined by squeezing the joint at the distal tibia and fibula. Plantar fasciitis and a heel spur may sometimes cause heel tenderness.

Ankle examination checklist

Inspection standing	• weight bearing • walking • swelling • Achilles' tendon
Inspection supine	• Achilles' tendon
Palpation	• Achilles' tendon • sinus tarsi • swelling, tenderness • bony survey, pulses • tendons
Movements	• active and passive
Ligaments	• collaterals
Anterior drawer test	

Ankle sprain

This is perhaps the most common sporting injury presenting to the family doctor. The typical ankle sprain occurs as a result of a forced inversion of the ankle. This action stresses the anterior talofibular ligament initially but with greater inversion forces may also stress the calcaneofibular ligament and the posterior talofibular ligaments. Pain and swelling occur first, with bruising later. Severe ankle injuries are usually seen at the accident and emergency department, and those presenting to the family doctor are often moderate to mild. If acting as the team doctor it may be possible to supervise immediate treatment but in any case athletes and officials should be aware of the appropriate first aid treatment. The priority is first aid with application of ice, compression and elevation. If ice is unavailable the next best option may be to put the foot in a bucket of cool water, or under the cold tap. The aim of this phase is to reduce bleeding and swelling. Current practice is to advise early mobilisation and to try to get the athlete to walk normally as soon as possible. Compression helps reduce swelling so ideally the patient would wear a compression bandage overnight and try to get the foot elevated as soon as possible.

More commonly the athlete presents to the surgery a day or so after the injury with a painful swollen ankle and bruising tracking down laterally, often to the lateral side of the foot. The sequence of rehabilitation is as follows.

Treatment
This is rest, ice, compression and elevation. Non-steroidal anti-inflammatory medication can help reduce pain, swelling and the inflammatory reaction and early physiotherapy may include ultrasound.

Rehabilitation
Early mobilisation of the ankle is the first stage in rehabilitation. With an acute injury the patient may be unable to weight bear but mobilisation can be carried out sitting using simple movements, such as drawing their name with their foot. Gentle passive stretching can help but not if it causes any pain. Resume muscle activity with isometric strengthening initially. This can be done by contracting the muscle against a fixed surface. Later isotonic exercise may be included using rolls of elastic cord or Cliniband (Figure 13.2).

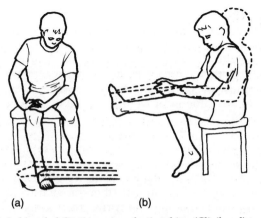

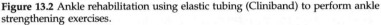

(a)   (b)

Figure 13.2 Ankle rehabilitation using elastic tubing (Cliniband) to perform ankle strengthening exercises.

Physiotherapists may use heat, massage and various electrical treatments. Proprioceptive training is perhaps the most important part of rehabilitation in the prevention of future injury. This is usually undertaken by the physiotherapist using a wobble board.

Exercise

Exercise should introduce progressive dynamic movements. Having achieved the first phase of rehabilitation the next stage is to begin progressive exercises such as jogging, running, swimming and cycling. One may also begin strengthening exercises and continue with stretching.

Activity

While the previous phase concentrated on non-specific activity the next phase is about getting back to all the movements associated with the sport. For ball players and all field sports it is essential to regain all the typical movements of the game before returning to competition. Before turning and changing direction at speed, the player must begin by jogging in straight lines with stopping to turn, gradually increasing the speed and reducing the arc of the turns. Full sprinting, jumping and return to all the non-competitive activities of the sport include sprinting, turning, cutting, and all changes of direction.

Target

The target is a return to competitive sport. It is essential to include a preventive strategy to avoid recurrence of the injury. This means pre-activity warm-up, stretching, the use of protective heat retaining clothes with post-activity warm-down, and exercise programmes to strengthen both agonists and antagonists. Taping may be of value in prevention of ankle sprains in certain sports.

Early mobilisation is the key, aiming for rapid return to weight-bearing exercise. In the second phase we aim for more sports-specific exercise. Once the patient can weight bear we begin with gentle jogging in straight lines, then move towards running in straight lines but walking the turns, then jogging the turns gently, and finally running in large semicircles. When an athlete can run and turn rapidly then he or she may return to proper training. Rehabilitation is sports specific and cyclists or rowers can often return to their sport much earlier than runners or field sports players as these sports do not require great functional movement at the ankle joint, and re-injury is unlikely. After an ankle sprain a cyclist or rower can return to their sport within days, while a track athlete may require 1 week, and a footballer, who must be able to run, cut, change direction and jump and land on an uneven pitch may take 10 days for full functional and proprioceptive rehabilitation.

Strapping the ankle

The purpose in early strapping is to provide compression and support. If there is gross swelling and pain then an elasticated support is most suitable. The most effective strapping for stability is the weave of adhesive bandage around the ankle and foot with a horseshoe of orthopaedic felt around the malleolus. Strapping may also help proprioception.

The Achilles' tendon

The Achilles' tendon is arguably the most important biomechanical link in sport. Injury to this tendon has a major effect on performance and achievement. Injury may be the classic overuse type picture with pain and inflammation or may be a sudden catastrophic rupture. From the athlete's perspective these injuries are equally important.

The tendon itself is made up of bands of collagen, with very little elastic component. The fibres of the tendon are rotated through 90° along the length of the tendon. This is a key feature in the aetiology of injury as recurrent ankle flexion and extension, as in distance running, can produce a sawing movement leading to degeneration. These foci of tissue degeneration may form nodules within the tendon which in turn weaken the tendon making it more susceptible to rupture. It may also lead to chronic pain and inflammation within the tendon.

Achilles' tendinitis has well recognised clinical features. At first the symptoms are mild and the athlete describes pain and stiffness in the morning which eases through the day. The pain and stiffness may be more noticeable when driving or after moving about after rest. In the early stages the athlete usually continues to train. The pain is at its worst in the initial part of training, in the first few miles of a run for example, but usually eases during the training session. The cycle of pain and inflammation begins again the next morning. There are many possible aetiological factors. Overuse is the key common factor, but Achilles' tendinitis does not occur in all those training intensely so there are other factors. It may be as a result of a biomechanical abnormality that the athlete puts excessive strain on the tendon. A runner who hyper-pronates, for example, puts excessive stretch and rotation on the Achilles' tendon causing tissue degeneration. Worn shoes, or pressure from the heel tab on the shoe may also add to the problem. Treatment is conservative and symptomatic while trying to eliminate the cause. A biomechanical abnormality may be modified using orthotics, either as internal shoe inserts, or by modifying the shoe by rebuilding with a mid sole wedge. Some shoes are manufactured to reduce pronation using wedge inserts in the sole. Modifying training by changing to a different surface, such as running on grass or softer surfaces reduce ground force. Reducing training mileage may also help. Some physiotherapists strongly advocate deep friction massage, and there are theoretical advantages to this treatment as it may reduce adhesions and increase blood flow. There is little scientific evidence, however, and deep friction massage can be extremely painful. Non-steroidal anti-inflammatory agents can reduce symptoms and reduce local inflammation. Steroid injections should be avoided. The Achilles' tendon requires considerable tensile strength. There is evidence that steroid injections may cause tissue degeneration and this may lead to Achilles' tendon rupture.

Achilles' tendon rupture

Rupture of the achilles tendon occurs suddenly and is often described as like a blow to the leg. It occurs, interestingly, more often on the left side and in men. It occurs in the older athlete, suggesting that there is an age-related tissue degeneration. Diagnosis is through history confirmed by examination. The history is classic. The patient describes a very sudden pain in the leg which is of such sudden and severe onset that they feel as if they were struck or kicked. This sudden snap leaves them with a weak ankle and they often limp into the accident and emergency department. Examination usually confirms the diagnosis. There is swelling and bruising and if the swelling is not extensive there may be a palpable defect in the tendon. If the diagnosis is still not clear a number of clinical tests are described which help confirm the diagnosis: these include Thompson's or Simmond's test. This test is carried out with the patient prone. When the Achilles' tendon is intact, squeezing the calf should produce plantar flexion at the ankle but this does not occur with a rupture. Diagnosis can be confirmed using the more modern radiological techniques of ultrasound and MRI.

There are two major schools of thought in management: surgical or conservative management with no clear evidence that one method is superior. Surgery is complicated by the difficulties of suturing the two ends of the tendon together as the ends may be quite frayed and the tendon is under constant tension and re-rupture is common. The skin incision is in an area of poor skin circulation and often healing is slow, with the risk of wound breakdown. Even after surgery, the ankle is fully immobilised for 6 weeks, although more recently partially articulating braces have been used. Conservative treatment is with cast immobilisation. The expert view is that, notwithstanding the complication rate, surgical management is best for the active athlete [3].

The chronic ankle sprain

The typical story is of the occasional athlete who has not played for months because their ankle 'does not feel right'. This patient requires a detailed examination and assessment by a physiotherapist. There may be a mechanical instability due to persistent ligamentous laxity and the ligaments should be assessed in detail. This should involve assessment of inversion, eversion and a drawer test. If there is excessive laxity causing instability the patient should have an orthopaedic assessment and occasionally surgery is necessary.

There may not, however, be ligament laxity and the feeling of insecurity may be due to other causes including persistent proprioception impairment. Retraining, proprioceptive exercises and taping may help non-mechanical ankle instability and are best undertaken by a skilled physiotherapist.

References

1 Bollen SR., Scott C. Rupture of the anterior cruciate ligament – a quiet epidemic? *Injury.* 1996; 27: 407–9.
2 O'Neill D. Arthroscopically assisted reconstruction of the anterior cruciate ligament. A prospective randomized analysis of three techniques. *J Bone Jt Surg* 1996; **78** [A]: 803–13.
3 Waterson SW, Mafulli N, Ewen SWB. Subcutaneous rupture of the Achilles' tendon: basic science and some aspects of clinical practice. *Br J Sports Med* 1997; **31**: 285–298.

14 Injuries of the foot

The foot is involved in almost every sporting activity, whether acting as a pivot, shock absorber or spring, or when used in kicking, gripping or to maintain balance. It is surprising perhaps that it is not injured more often. Even during a 30 minute run the foot withstands thousands of impacts, each with a force of more than three times body weight. The foot is also the first link in the lower limb kinetic chain so that injuries of the foot affect the forces and biomechanical balance of the entire leg. It has a key role as a shock absorber, mediated particularly through the two main arches: the longitudinal and transverse arch. Damage to these structures increases impact stress which is transmitted upwards leading to problems in the foot, ankle, leg and hip. Sport-related foot problems which are common in general practice include stress fractures, turf toe and tendinitis. Other common general practice problems include skin conditions and athletes foot.

Stress fractures

Stress fractures can occur, usually in the metatarsals. The so-called march fracture of the 2nd metatarsal is a stress fracture, but stress fractures can occur in any of the metatarsals and indeed many of the weight-bearing foot bones. The diagnosis may be made by X-ray in the later stages and in the early stages by bone scan. As with all stress fractures, the treatment is rest but sometimes a plaster cast is necessary for immobilisation. Stress fractures of the metatarsals can usually be treated in general practice but stress fractures of the other foot bones, in particular the navicular, may require specialist supervision.

Plantar fasciitis

Plantar fasciitis is a common general practice problem. It used attract the title 'policeman's heel' at a time when policemen walked the beat. Exercise is usually the cause, and it is a typical overuse injury. The athlete presents with persistent heel pain with the point of greatest tenderness just at the anterior margin of the heel pad. The pain is usually most severe in the morning or when walking after periods of rest. Sometimes there is a precipitating cause, perhaps a change of training terrain, different running shoes, or an additional activity such as climbing ladders while decorating. An X-ray may show a heel spur, although the absence of any finding on X-ray is unlikely to alter treatment.

There are two main parts to treatment. The first is in modifying the traction on the fascia. This can be achieved by using a heel pad. Commercially available pads are suitable, although orthopaedic felt can suffice. Stretching should theoretically help but the exercises are difficult. A splint which stretches the plantar fascia at night has theoretical benefit. The second part of treatment is in reducing the local inflammation. Ultrasound, anti-inflammatory medication and anti-inflammatory gel can help, but eventually a corticosteroid injection may be required. The injection can be painful but is usually effective. It is better to avoid surgery if at all possible and a heel spur does not indicate a need for surgery. This condition is best managed conservatively.

Pain at the posterior heel, at the insertion of the Achilles' tendon may be a traction apophysitis or Sever's disease. This condition is usually treated conservatively.

Impact heel

Runners and other athletes who strike the ground hard with their heel may develop chronic heel pain. This may be due to inflammation of the heel fat pad. When this occurs it is very difficult to treat. Inflammation is reduced with rest but often recurs when the athlete goes back to sport. The only effective treatment is to reduce the heel impact using a heel insert.

Flexor tendinitis

Pain on the dorsum of the foot may be due to inflammation of the tendons. This is often due to pressure from the laces or the tongue of the shoe on the dorsum of the foot. Topical anti-inflammatory medication helps, but the problem is often easily cured by loosening or changing the shoe lacing.

Hyperpronation

If a patient tells you that they hyperpronate what do they mean? All running shoe shops and many runners use the term hyperpronation. It describes exaggerated eversion of the foot that may occur during the weight-bearing and take-off phase of running.

In the normal gait, the foot strikes the ground with the heel first. As weight is taken, the outer border of the foot makes contact with the ground and as more weight is taken the foot flattens out and the arch of the foot flattens taking the strain. The foot thus acts as a dynamic shock absorber on foot strike. If the foot is pronated excessively during this phase of foot strike the shock absorbing effect is impaired. With a foot that is too flat, or hyperpronated, there is increased transmission of impact up through the leg and there is also a rotation of the tibia. This altered dynamic posture may give rise to many different problems including Achilles' tendonitis, stress fractures, compartment syndromes and patellofemoral pain. By altering the biomechanics of foot strike it is possible to minimise hyperpronation. One may use shoe inserts or orthotics, or may buy shoes specially designed to minimise pronation. These are available from a number of manufacturers and usually include an alteration to the sole of the shoe and reinforcement of the uppers. Many runners have a hyperpronated gait and suffer few problems, so hyperpronation does not necessarily need to be treated unless it causes symptoms. Those who hyperpronate should be advised, however, that their natural shock absorbing dynamics may be impaired and they should wear good quality shoes with adequate shock absorption and try, where possible, to run on a forgiving surface. The diagnosis is usually made on observation of the athlete running when exaggerated eversion can be seen. If hyperpronation is severe the foot may appear flat on standing. A further diagnostic test is to observe the angle made by the Achilles' tendon in the half squat. Hyperpronation in not a disease or medical condition, it is an altered dynamic posture which may give problems in some athletes but not all. There is little evidence that treating asymptomatic athletes can prevent problems.

Fractures

Fractures of the foot can occasionally be missed at accident and emergency and sometimes present in general practice as persistent pain. One of the fractures to look out for is a fracture of the 5th metatarsal. Pain and tenderness can persist after injury and this fracture can persist to non-union. Referral for X-ray and, if a fracture is detected, a plaster cast with orthopaedic referral is appropriate.

Turf toe

The so-called turf toe is an injury to the first metatarsalphalangeal joint (MTP joint). It usually occurs when the foot is caught awkwardly, spraining the joint. It can occur with hyperextension or flexion. It is painful, uncomfortable and can make sport difficult. Strapping can help in the short term and the joint usually recovers without significant problems. If the toe is very painful an X-ray is appropriate to exclude a fracture.

Abnormal feet

Athletes seem to be able to compete happily with the most unusual feet. Unless they are causing problems these abnormalities are best ignored. Athletes often have bunions, hallux valgus, hammer toes and skin calluses but they are asymptomatic. They have often found a shoe or insole or a means of protecting the foot that solves the problem. In most of these cases medical intervention is inappropriate.

Other common problems of the foot that may require treatment are interdigital neuromas, inflammation of the sesamoid bones and metatarsalgia. Neuromas occur when the interdigital nerve is bruised causing pain and tingling along the distribution of the nerve. The treatment is rest. Problems may arise with the sesamoid bones under the big toe. They are best treated by rest and suitable pressure-relieving insoles; surgery is best avoided.

Occasionally, if they cause persistent problems through fractures or inflammation, surgery may be justified although recovery is not always straightforward and the long-term outcome may not be satisfactory.

Metatarsalgia causes a pain across the head of the metatarsal. It is usually due to a change in shoes or increase in training. Treatment is by relieving the pressure on the metatarsal head, using an orthopaedic felt insert. The insert should be proximal to the metatarsal head thus reducing the pressure. If the insert is under the metatarsal heads, this simply increases the pressure on the bone.

Footwear

Sports footwear can provoke many problems. One of the most common general practice problems are the dermatological hazards from wearing running or training shoes continuously. Other problems arise from wearing the wrong shoe, for the wrong sport, or on the wrong surface.

Running shoes are made for running and usually have a raised heel and a thick shock absorbing sole. They are made for running in straight lines forward and have sharp edges at the sides of the sole and heel. Indoor training or cross-training shoes are made for rotation movements and have rounded edges to their soles. If someone plays indoor games on a running shoe, they are at risk of 'falling off' the shoe by catching the sharp angle as they try to change direction.

There is also the suggestion that the design of some running shoes may exacerbate Achilles' tendinitis. Many shoes are built up at the back with a heel tab at the Achilles' tendon. On plantar flexion this heel tab impinges on the tendon and may cause pain. Those with Achilles' tendon pain would be advised to cut off the offending heel tab.

When buying a sports shoe, athletes would be well advised to seek help in a specialised sports shoe store. They must buy a shoe that is correct for their sport and correct for them. If the buyer is 90 kg with poor running technique, they need a well supported shoe with adequate shock absorption. The most appropriate model will not be the same as that designed for the 55 kg elite marathon runner who glides along the surface. If they hyperpronate, they may benefit from a shoe specially designed for this condition or if they have Achilles' tendinitis they may be better with shoe that has a low heel tab.

When a patient with sports-related lower limb pain attends with a problem they should be asked to bring their sports shoe with them. Sometimes the diagnosis can be made from examination of the shoe.

15 Taping and injection

Taping and strapping have been used by generations of sports medicine physicians and physiotherapists. It has become so much a part of the ritual in some sports that to question its value is heresy. Logically, one could not expect adhesive strapping to prevent an ankle inversion injury by resisting the momentum of a 15 stone footballer running at 15 m.p.h. Strapping small joints may help resist applied forces but the benefits gained by strapping larger joints could not be due the strength of the tape alone. The answer may be through its effect in augmenting proprioception.

A recent review [1] of the role of taping and bracing in the athlete concluded that both the mechanical and functional stability of the ankle can be improved with taping. Taping with zinc oxide tape certainly provides some mechanical stability [2,3] but the effect is short term. Clearly the benefit is greater than that gained from mechanical stability alone and this review suggests that neuromuscular and sensory factors contribute greatly. It seems that some of the benefits of strapping are mediated by the peroneal muscles. Taping is of benefit in prevention and in treatment of the injured ankle but ankle bracing also has a role as braces can exert mechanical restriction of ankle movement for longer and may also have some proprioceptive effect.

Taping

Taping methods are shown in Figures 15.1, 15.2, 15.3 and 15.4.

Injection technique

Most simple local inflammatory sports medicine conditions are within the remit of the general practitioner. In many cases injury

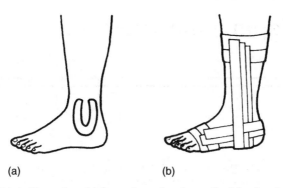

(a)   (b)

Figure 15.1 Ankle taping: (a) horseshoe of orthopaedic felt placed around the lateral malleolus and (b) lateral stirrups or basketweave taping to prevent inversion of the ankle.

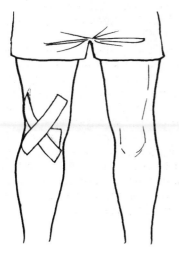

Figure 15.2 Patella taping for anterior knee pain. A diagonal strip is applied from the lower lateral aspect pulling proximally across the patellar tendon and ending medially.

can be treated using simple physical methods together with the appropriate modification of training and alteration in technique. Occasionally, chronic inflammatory conditions may require local injection of corticosteroid. Injection should be seen as an adjunct to other aspects of management which includes identifying the cause of the injury and modification of training or technique.

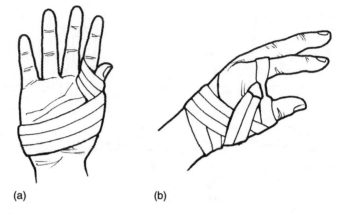

Figure 15.3 Taping for injury to the ulnar collateral ligament of the thumb.

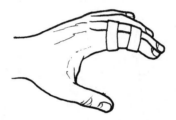

Figure 15.4 Buddy taping' fixes the injured finger to its neighbour.

General practitioners are often anxious about injections. There are well recognised hazards. Infection is always a risk, so one should always use an aseptic technique. Corticosteroid may impair the local body response to infection which adds to the risk. An injection should never be given if there is local skin infection or if there is any possibility of prior septic arthritis. Other recognised side-effects include atrophy of soft tissue, skin discoloration due to depigmentation, and tissue degeneration. In general these side-effects are due to poor technique or use of too large a dose but they are often unpredictable. Tendon rupture can occur due to the catabolic effect of the steroid on collagen, so an injection should never be made into the tendon. For this reason most general practitioners avoid injecting major weight-bearing tendons such as the patella or Achilles' tendon. Care should also be taken to avoid the median nerve in carpal tunnel injection and the ulnar nerve in injection of golfer's elbow at the medial epicondyle. In general, it is ill advised to perform intrarticular joint injections in young athletes. It is always important to warn patients of the risks of injections and to document this on the medical record.

A corticosteroid injection is usually given together with local anaesthetic. When the local anaesthetic wears off, usually in a few hours, there may be some local pain. This pain may increase in severity over the next 12–24 hours. This secondary pain is a reaction to the microcrystals which make up the corticosteroid suspension and is similar to the crystalline reaction that occurs in gout. It may be 24–48 hours before the corticosteroid injection begins to exert an anti-inflammatory effect. It is accepted practice that one does not inject any inflammatory lesion more than three times or a joint more than once. These rules are more empirical than based on evidence, and reflect doctors' anxiety about the catabolic effect of corticosteroid.

Corticosteroids are available in a number of formulations. A summary of the preparations, the risks and precautions was recently published in the *Drug and Therapeutics Bulletin* [4]. Hydrocortisone acetate, introduced 40 years ago, was the first to be used and there are now seven corticosteroids licensed for use. The dose is usually determined by the size of the joint. Hydrocortisone acetate (Hydrocortistab) has a weak anti-inflammatory effect but it is relatively soluble and is absorbed quickly. Longer acting preparations include methylprednisolone (Depomedrone), triamcinolone (Adcortyl, Lederspan) and prednisolone acetate (Deltastab). These are about five times more potent, are much less soluble and are longer acting. These medications may have more than a local effect with possible suppression of the hypothalamic–pituitary-adrenal axis.

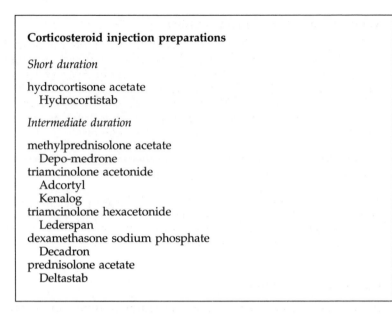

Corticosteroid injection preparations

Short duration

hydrocortisone acetate
　Hydrocortistab

Intermediate duration

methylprednisolone acetate
　Depo-medrone
triamcinolone acetonide
　Adcortyl
　Kenalog
triamcinolone hexacetonide
　Lederspan
dexamethasone sodium phosphate
　Decadron
prednisolone acetate
　Deltastab

Where and how to inject

Such injections should be given adhering to proper aseptic technique. There should be adequate skin preparation with cleansing and the doctor should use gloves and a no-touch technique. The doctor should be familiar with injection technique, know the anatomy well, and use the correct sized needle and local anaesthetic. By convention, no more than three injections are given to any one site in a year.

After steroid injection the patient should rest for 48 hours. This means avoidance of exercise of the injected part and that includes heavy lifting or carrying. If they have a manual occupation the injection should be performed at a time when they have an opportunity to rest. For patients with rheumatoid arthritis or osteoarthritis, a longer acting corticosteroid preparation is probably of more benefit. In most sports-related injuries the aim of the injection is to stop the pain and inflammation cycle so that the technique can be modified or training altered to eliminate the problem. A shorter duration preparation may be appropriate because of the reduced potential for long-term side-effects, tissue catabolism and tendon rupture.

Tennis elbow (lateral epicondylitis)

In this injection we infiltrate the junction between the muscle and its attachment to bone. Infiltrate around the tender area with 2–5 ml (approx. 20 mg hydrocortisone acetate or 5 mg of triamcinolone with 1% lignocaine). Sometimes tennis elbow does not respond to the first injection and may require two–three injections. If the condition does not respond after three injections one should perhaps think again about the diagnosis.

Golfer's elbow (medial epicondylitis)

This condition has a similar aetiology and treatment but many general practitioners are concerned about injecting around the medial epicondyle because of the proximity of the ulnar nerve in the groove just behind the epicondyle.

Carpal tunnel syndrome

An unusual sports-related injury although common in general practice. It is usual to confirm the diagnosis before injection. The symptoms occur due to medial nerve compression beneath the flexor retinaculum. The symptoms are mostly sensory with numbness and parasthesia of the median nerve distribution to the palmar surface of the index, middle and medial side of the ring finger although these symptoms are often proximally too. Tinel's sign is where tapping the median nerve at the wrist reproduces the symptoms.

The injection is in the middle of the wrist, just lateral to the tendon of palmaris longus and medial to flexor carpi radialis. Inject at the line of the crease between wrist and hand. The injection volume should be about 1 ml (approx. 10 mg of hydrocortisone acetate or 3 mg of triamcinolone with 1% lignocaine) using a fine bore needle.

Tenosynovitis

This is a common sports injury that responds well to injection. Inject tangentially along the line of the tendon, but not into the tendon. It should be possible to inject into the synovial sheath without resistance and palpate the injection in the sheath (approx 10 mg of hydrocortisone acetate or 3 mg of triamcinolone with 1% lignocaine made up to 2 ml).

Shoulder

The acromioclavicular joint may be injected using a fine needle (approx 2 mg of triamcinolone with 1% lignocaine made up to 0.5 ml).

Injection of a painful arc can have good results in subacromial bursitis. The approach is lateral, or a little posterior to the lateral position aiming to insert the needle below the acromium into the subacromial space. The needle is introduced pointing upwards toward the ear. There should be little resistance to injection. A larger volume of fluid is injected (approx 20–40 mg of hydrocortisone acetate or 10–20 mg of triamcinolone depending on the size of the patient with 1% lignocaine made up to 5 ml).

Trochanteric bursitis

The area of tenderness is usually over the greater trochanter. With the patient lying sideways on the couch, identify the area of tenderness and infiltrate widely. Using local anaesthetic and corticosteroid (approx 20 mg of hydrocortisone acetate or 5 mg of triamcinolone with 1% lignocaine made up to 5 ml).

Prepatellar bursitis

It may be possible to aspirate the bursa, although not always possible if the bursa has loculated. Injection of a small quantity of hydrocortisone can help reduce the bursa and prevent recurrence (approx 5 mg of hydrocortisone acetate with 1% lignocaine).

Iliotibial band

On the lateral side of the knee where the iliotibial band crosses the lateral femoral condyle (approx 5 mg of hydrocortisone acetate with 1% lignocaine made up to 2 ml).

Pes anserinus bursitis

Inject the medial side of the knee at the pes anserinus insertion (approx 5 mg of hydrocortisone acetate with 1% lignocaine made up to 2 ml).

Plantar fasciitis (policeman's heel)

This is a painful injection from the medial side. The tissue is quite tight and only a small volume may be injected (approx 2 mg of triamcinolone with 1% lignocaine made up to 0.5 ml).

Rheumatologists and orthopaedic surgeons inject many other joints with considerable success. For the general practitioner with an interest in sport and physical medicine who is not regularly injecting joints, it is reasonable to begin with these few basic injections and to progress with expert tuition. The instructions above are suitable for those who can remember their anatomy. If you cannot quite remember where the structures are I suggest that you look for one of the texts on detailed injection technique [5–7].

References

1 Callaghan MJ. Role of ankle taping and bracing in the athlete. *Br J Sports Med* 1997; **31**: 102–8.
2 Rarick GL, Bigley G, Karst P, Malina RM. The measurable support of the ankle joint by conventional methods of taping. *J Bone Jt Surg* 1962; **44** [A]: 1183–90.
3 Frankley JR, Jewett DL, Hanks GA, Sebastianelli WJ. A comparison of ankle tape methods. *Clin J Sport Med* 1993; **3**: 20–5.
4 Articular and periarticular corticosteroid injections. *Drug Therap Bull* 1995; **33**: 67–70.
5 Austin K, Gwynn-Brett K, Marshall S. *Illustrated Guide to Taping Techniques.* Wolfe, London, 1994.
6 Saunders S, Cameron G. *Injection Techniques in Orthopaedic and Sports Medicine.* Saunders, London, 1997.
7 StJ Dixon, Graber J. *Local Injection Therapy in Rheumatic Diseases.* Eular, Basle, 1989.

16 The team doctor

Many of us are just a phone call away from becoming a team doctor. The responsibility can vary from chief medical officer of a major national sporting organisation to giving medical advice on your child's ski trip. The scale may be different but the basic principles are the same.

It is unlikely that you will be asked to become medical officer to a national sporting body without long involvement with that sport. You are more likely to have been involved as a participant at first and to have gradually become more involved in a professional capacity. From this background you will have experience and expertise and knowledge of the sport. Perhaps the most important attribute is the knowledge of the particular problems of that sport because the roles of medical officers can be very varied and quite challenging: the doctor at an athletics event may never leave the medical room, while the doctor on a major cycling race may be asked to administer first aid from the window of a car at 25 miles per hour. The doctor on a cricket tour has a very different role to that of doctor on a ocean racing yacht. Similarly the doctors providing medical cover at a boxing competition, rugby match or tennis tournament will have very different roles. If a doctor acts as drug control officer, the role and responsibilities are very different again. There is, in addition, a new type of sports doctor known as the 'crowd doctor', whose brief is not to look after incidents on the field of play but to care for the spectators.

The doctor's responsibilities

As team doctor your responsibility is always to your patient, but this role may vary according to the circumstances and conditions of employment. There are times when there may be a conflict between your duty to the team and to the individual. It is important to clarify with both the player and the management where the prime responsibility lies. If employed by a team or organisation there is a parallel between the role of the team doctor and that of an occupational health physician where the duty to a team may override a patient's wish to hide an injury. It is essential that doctor, patient and management know exactly where the lines of responsibility begin and end and which role the doctor is undertaking at any particular time.

You may come under pressure from management, and perhaps from the press, to discuss confidential matters between you and the player but your duty of care is still to the player. You may be asked to adjudicate as to a player's fitness, a decision that is not always without controversy. Clearly a fitness test is a matter between the player, the doctor, the physiotherapist and the coach but there may be occasions when the doctor's opinion is not in agreement with the wishes of the manager or indeed the player who wants to play.

As doctor to a national governing body, you may be asked to adjudicate on matters of health and safety, an aspect of sport that is poorly developed and where few guidelines are available [1]. You may be asked for advice on safety issues, for example on the need for cycle helmets, if a jockey is fit to compete after recovery from injury, or on the safety of certain medications.

The doctor on a training camp has yet a different role with responsibilities for both treatment and prevention. At the training camp, the management of medical problems may not be so acute but you may perhaps be asked to undertake screening medical examinations. The purpose of such examination is to screen for potential medical problems that could recur at later, more critical, moments in a season. During a training camp there may be an opportunity to give advice on diet, stretching, injury prevention and other health care issues. It also provides a forum for discussion of problems of drug abuse and the risk of possible inadvertent drug positives.

Looking after a major event

The best medical involvement is no involvement. Not that there should be neglect of the medical needs of participants in a major event, but the advice to participants and preparation of both participants and medical services should be such that there is either no need, or that services work so efficient and seamlessly that their presence is not noticed. As with every sporting event the most important people are the participants and medical services are only there in support.

There are a number of key factors which range from the logistical and organisational to the care of the individual patient. In planning and organisation of services, preparation should begin at the earliest moment, working closely with the organising committee. For a mass participation event the medical team should begin by profiling the type of person they expect to participate. Details of the preparation required by a medical team in preparation for such an event have been published previously and those invited to act as medical officer for a mass participation event are advised to consult the original article in the British Medical Journal [2]. The upsurge of marathon running brought us an awareness that not all those competing, even in an event so challenging as a marathon, will be fit and healthy. For example there are many reasons for undertaking a marathon and many cardiac, respiratory or renal transplant patients regard completing such an event as a validation of their health. Some participants are poorly prepared and while their intentions were good when they submitted their application their training programme never came to fruition. Allowing participants to defer their entry until the following year can help reduce the pressure on participants to compete if their entry has been accepted but they have not adequately prepared. One can seldom predict the weather and one can never depend on our climate. The organising committee must decide at the earliest point how they are to plan for problems.

Ideally those at risk should be identified from the entry form. Many mass participation events ask applicants to state if they have any health problems but applicants may not tell the whole truth fearing that they may be excluded, so it must be clear that medical details are for planning only and not for exclusion. Asking participants to sign a fitness declaration is no guarantee of good health or preparation. At the event itself the medical team would ideally have some means of identifying those with medical problems, either from printed details on the reverse of the number, or from a medical history written on their number. This is not foolproof as participants may swap numbers, lose their number or not include details. Some participants may feel that it is an intrusion or stigma to suggest that medical factors are important and that their health is their concern alone.

In order to minimise health crises there are a number of possible precautions one may take. When people enter such an event they may be sent a medical advice leaflet with their entry confirmation suggesting when and how participants can withdraw, and indicate why they should not participate if feeling unwell on the day of the event. In order to encourage participants to be adequately prepared one may include a training plan and suggest minimal levels of preparation or fitness. There will, however, always be those competing who are ill, inadequately prepared or simply not fit enough.

Precise environmental conditions cannot be planned although seasonal variations will give some idea of the expected temperature, humidity and wind chill. These will all affect planning. It may be inappropriate to allow the event to commence or continue in inappropriate environmental conditions.

With a large number of participants and spectators, there must be advance planning of first aid stations, ambulance services, medical, nursing, physiotherapy and other personnel, emergency equipment and transport arrangements to the hospitals. The local accident and emergency departments must be notified. It is important to coordinate the services of the voluntary bodies and their ambulance personnel. Volunteers acting as marshals on the marathon should also be considered part of the extended medical team and have a role in preventing medical problems. Fluid replacement stations should be available at strategic points and adequate quantity and variety of fluid should be available. The warm-down area must be well supervised and staffed by those who know how to deal with postexercise syncope, hyper- and hypothermia, and fluid replacement. There should also be an opportunity for participants to withdraw from the event at any stage with suitable transport arrangements back to the pick-up points. Encouraging or assisting those who are clearly unwell or suffering to continue at any part of the event is to be discouraged and every opportunity afforded to allow them to withdraw with honour. A doctor may be invited to provide medical care at a sporting event at relatively short notice and may not have been involved in planning. This can put the doctor in a very difficult position when expected to provide cover for an event where they have not been involved in planning the medical facilties or procedures for dealing with casualties.

Remember too, that this event may draw a large number of spectators and they may also have medical problems. It is important for follow-up of all casualties to be arranged and for the event doctor to be available for consultation by the media should any untoward medical event occur.

On the day of the event the doctor is far down the list of importance in the hierarchy of the back-room staff, except in a medical emergency when the doctor is expected to be able to cope with all eventualities. The ideal team doctor is unseen except when their services are required and at that moment should mysteriously appear highly prepared to cope with any possible emergency. It is unnecessary to become involved in minor injury, to make unnecessary incursions onto the field of play, or interrupt the sport. Some injuries are of course exaggerated for the benefit of the referee, or recovery delayed to seek time advantage and miracles seem to happen regularly on the sports field! The ideal event doctor knows exactly when they are needed, and when they are in the way.

The pre-participation medical examination

Patients often ask to have a 'medical' before they take up a sport, at the start of the season, or when they join a health club. Many sporting organisations encourage participants to have a pre-participation examination, and many lay articles on exercise promotion suggest that participants seek their doctor's advice before beginning. The value and indeed the appropriate content of this examination is debatable. The main purpose of such an examination is to exclude those who are physically unable to participate or who may be at risk from participation. This would include: detection of physical disabilities that would prevent participation, screening those at risk due to previously undetected medical conditions, ensuring that those with previously known medical conditions are not put at risk, and possible insurance requirements.

The history and examination are both general and specific but should have a particular focus depending on the nature of the proposed sport or activity. A example of a focused medical examination is the pre-participation diving examination, with its clearly presented criteria relating to examination of the ear, nose and throat and of the respiratory system.

Medical screening may include a questionnaire. The screening questionnaire may help focus medical history taking on important features such as hospital attendances or admissions or significant or serious illnesses. It should also record a full drug history and should ask specifically if the athlete has taken alternative medical therapies, vitamins or supplements that may, in the case of a competitive sport, contain prohibited medical substances. It is becoming increasingly important to ask about diet and nutrition.

The pre-participation sports examination should include a baseline general medical examination but the sport-specific medical examination is in more detail. Important problems that should be identified include hernias, impacted wisdom teeth, asthma, chronic infection etc. It is very important that these are picked up early so that, for example, dental treatment or hernia repair can be arranged early in the season and not cause team disruption at a critical point in the season. The musculoskeletal examination is of particular importance. In particular it is important to look for full free and unrestricted head and neck movements. The ENT examination should include examination of the tympanic membrane to detect perforation or discharge, and nasal deviation or discharge. Visual acuity and visual fields are important for certain sports. Examination of the mouth and teeth should exclude caries which could cause problems later in the season including impacted or partially erupted wisdom teeth.

In examination of the cardiovascular and respiratory system, it is important to detect reversible airways obstruction which may be remedial to treatment and help the athlete's performance. If suspected, an exercise stress test with spirometry may detect deterioration in peak flow rates. Cardiovascular examination should include auscultation of the heart for murmurs to detect hypertrophic obstructive cardiomyopathy (HOCM) in particular and blood pressure should be recorded. Examination of the abdomen should exclude organomegaly, hepato- or splenomegaly which may be vulnerable to trauma in contact sports. Examination of the hernial orifices is also essential. Skin conditions are often a problem in sport with bacterial or fungal infections. Examination of the musculoskeletal system should include a detailed examination of all joints for active and passive movements. Normal variants such as excessive kyphoscoliosis or pes planus can cause problems in some sports.

A detailed medical examination may include a physiological assessment. This physiological appraisal may include a large battery of tests or a selection of sport-specific tests from a wide menu. It is important to focus of the needs of the particular sport. A battery of tests with a generic threshold fitness level is inappropriate. Tests may not have functional implications. Reduced hearing, for example, is a disability but should not preclude someone from playing darts. Good cardiorespiratory endurance fitness is essential in a marathon runner but of lesser importance in a gymnast. Cruciate ligament instability may not impair performance in endurance sports such as cycling or rowing but would be critical in sports that require dynamic stability such as football. A physiological fitness test can have a specific use but should not be used indiscriminantly. It has sport-specific use only.

There is a perception amongst many of the general public that a medical examination is necessary before taking part in sport. Clearly, not everyone requires a physical examination. In recent major health and activity surveys, a random selection of the population in the UK exercised on a treadmill without specialist cardiac supervision. They used a pre-participation screening questionnaire help identify those who may have been unfit to undertake the appraisal. This pre-screening questionnaire focused specifically on cardiac, respiratory and functional limitations to exercise.

Pre-tour medical examination

Before major sporting events or before going to a major games you may be asked to perform pre-tour medical examinations. In many cases the organisation is spending a large amount of money in sending a team on tour and the doctor has a duty to ensure that all those travelling are fit. The team depends on each individual and the coach or management builds the team based on assumption that travelling players are fit and available for selection. If a player goes on tour, then someone else is always left behind and while one assumes that players only make themselves available if they are fit, this may not always be so. For this reason the doctor may have to examine players before departure. The main purpose of this examination is to ensure that no member of the team is carrying an injury or previously undiagnosed illness or ailment that could affect performance. At the very least, members of the touring party should complete a short questionnaire about current illness and past medical history. They should also list all medications, either prescribed or obtained elsewhere, and these should be reviewed in detail to ensure that they include only permitted medication. As any individual illness could affect the team's performance the doctor's responsibility in this situation is to the team. The divided loyalty of the doctor to both the individual and to the team should be clearly stated.

The pre-tour medical should also give the player the opportunity to discuss other possible health problems and gives the doctor a chance to record any past illness and anticipate any difficulties. The doctor should keep a permanent medical record in the same way as one would do in normal clinical practice. These records remain the property of the doctor and not of the player or management.

As general practitioners we routinely perform medical examinations for insurance companies, driving licences and such like and we are all aware of the limitations of clinical examination. It is not difficult for a player deliberately to disguise a minor current injury and the management may have unrealistic expectations of the examination. The doctor cannot be a fortune teller. But, in spite of the limitations of such examination, the doctor should adhere to a strict protocol. We have seen how this can be organised and regulated in the detailed clinical examination required of divers before they are issued with a licence, and this professional approach should be common to all sports.

The transfer medical

Performing the transfer medical of a player places the doctor in a very different position. In this situation the doctor's responsibility is to the club or organisation requesting the examination and his or her role is to find potential medical problems and to undertake appropriate investigations to ensure that no potential medical problems are missed.

The medical bag

Each travelling sports doctor has their own list of preferred medications and plans the content of their bag depending on the size of the team, their location, the ease of getting prescriptions locally and the expected workload. There is never enough space for everything you would like to bring, and someone will always ask for some simple and obvious medication or dressing that you have not brought. This following list is not comprehensive, but is to act as an *aide-memoire* which you may expand or ignore.

Contents of the team doctor's bag

Medications

Travel	Avomine
	temazepam
Pain relief	aspirin
	paracetamol
Anti-infective	amoxycillin
	erythromycin
	trimethoprim
	flucloxacillin
	metronidazole
Antifungal	topical antifungal agents
	vaginal medication if appropriate
Gastric	ranitidine
	Gaviscon
	Lomotil/imodium (NB enough for the team)
	Dioralyte
Local medications	Fluorescein
	chloromycetin
	local anaesthetic
	Aureocort (topical steroid/antibacterial)
	Cerumol
Asthma	inhalers
	nebuliser and medication (an appropriate attachment including travel adaptor)
Dressings	icepacks/cold sprays
	crêpe bandages
	gauze squares
	Tubigrip
	Elastoplast
	dressing packs
	eye patches
	Micropore
	Sofra-Tulle
	Melolin
	slings
	collar and cuff
	orthopaedic felt
Suture packs	lignocaine
	syringes 2 ml and 5 ml
	needles
	spirit/Savlon
	dressing pack/cotton wool
	suture material

▶

Taping	underwrap/zinc oxide tape (more than you think)
Equipment	opthalmoscope
	auroscope
	sphygmomanometer
	stethoscope
	tongue depressor
	forceps/tweezers/scissors/suture equipment
Skin preparations	topical antibacterials
	sun barriers
	moisturiser
	emergency medical bag

At the clubhouse

A telephone always available
Icepacks
Neck collars of various sizes
Splints
Stretcher, ideally a scoop
Airways
Laryngoscope and airways
Dripsets, needles and fluid

Legal responsibilities

Times have changed in general practice and all GPs are acutely aware of the medicolegal risks associated with practice. These changes are paralleled in sports medicine. With increasing knowledge and teaching available in sport and exercise medicine, athletes in all sports expect a high level of professional expertise from those caring for them. The day of the glorious amateur, providing medical advice on the touchline without relevant knowledge and expertise, should be gone. Accepting a post of medical adviser, even an honorary position, creates the expectation of a level of knowledge and expertise. If a doctor accepts a post as medical officer or similar position the legal expectation is that they have the knowledge and expertise similar to the standard of any doctor in that role [3]. They may be asked to show evidence of expertise and continued education and training in that field just as if they were providing paediatric or obstetric care.

The contract need not be written, the agreement to provide care is in itself a declaration of acceptance of the responsibility and the expected level of knowledge that goes with it. It is insufficient to state that there is no monetary value. In any case, most medical officers benefit from at least free attendance, privileged seats or an invitation to the club dinner. The contract need not be monetary or its equivalent, the contract is the acceptance of the role and the expectations that go with it. The 'good Samaritan' need not fear however. A doctor who happens to be attending an event, providing they have not been asked to act as a medical officer or have not accepted responsibility to act in a medical capacity, can give medical advice on a first aid basis. They would be well advised, however, not to exceed their duty of responsibility.

For GPs who provide medical advice in the surgery the situation is slightly different. Doctors advise people to be active, in keeping with accepted medical practice. They should have some knowledge of the risks and benefits of exercise but the level of expertise expected is that of any GP and not specialist knowledge. The rule of thumb is the Bolam rule [4] which infers that the care given should be of a level and expertise usually provided by a responsible body of medical opinion. A GP giving advice in the normal course of practice on matters relating to sport and exercise medicine would only be expected to have knowledge similar to that of other GPs.

If someone accepts a position of medical officer or medical adviser in sport, they are implicitly accepting a higher level of responsibility and would be expected to have a greater level of expertise. Now that well developed programmes of education and professional qualifications are available in sport and exercise medicine there is little excuse for lack of knowledge.

The MacLeod guidelines

MacLeod sets out the role and responsibilities of doctors who undertake responsibilities in sport and exercise medicine [5].

- Know the rules of the game and the recognised injury and illness patterns of the game or event.
- Clarify relationships with players, management, media and sponsors.
- Clarify responsibilities for crowd control and drug testing.
- Establish a good records system, which may range from pre-participation medical examinations to documentation of injury events and rehabilitation programmes.

- Identify and minimise risk, i.e. in the climatic and playing environment.
- Ensure that appropriate, qualified and insured personnel as well as facilities for treatment and support, rescue, first aid, transport to hospital and communications are available.
- Prepare yourself in professional terms for responsibilities equivalent to an appointment to a post in an A&E Department combined with a physically and psychologically demanding 'industry' i.e. sport.
- Join an appropriate specialty association and attend the relevant training programme.
- Ensure that you are adequately insured, especially if you are not a general practitioner.
- The doctor/patient relationship and player safety must remain your principal concern. Do no harm and minimise the risk of harm.

GPs may also be concerned about their responsibility in respect of staff who give advice on their behalf. A recent editorial [6] by a representative of one of the medical defence bodies clarified this issue. If the advice is given by a member of the employed staff, then the employee can expect to be protected by the employer for claims of damage, thus the doctor is responsible. If the doctor refers a patient to a fitness instructor or gymnasium, then the doctor is expected to have taken some reasonable steps to ensure that the referral is to a reputable and properly qualified instructor or organisation. Of course the doctor should counsel the patient and advise on aspects of the medical history that may have a bearing on the ability to exercise, and the risks.

The doctor is also expected to conform to the standards of ethical and professional integrity as set out by the General Medical Council. This is an important issue in the context of top level international sport where doctors may be under huge press and public pressure to breach confidentiality.

Sport and exercise medicine is developing as a discipline and with these changes are additional responsibilities. In particular there are additional medicolegal responsibilities. The usual medicolegal and ethical responsibilities still stand of course, and in keeping with normal practice a doctor should adhere to the normal ethical guidelines, treat to the best of their ability and record everything.

Medical screening

Medical screening questionnaires are provided by the Federation Internationale de Medecine Sportive (FIMS). Many other organisations such as the Australian Institute of Sport, Scottish Sports

Medicine Institute, British Olympic Association and the American College of Cardiology have their own guidelines.

References

1 Fuller CW, Hawkins R. Developing a health surveillance strategy for professional footballers in compliance with UK health and safety legislation. *Br J Sports Med* 1997; **31**: 148–151.
2 Popular marathons, half marathons and other long distance runs; recommendations for medical support. *BMJ* 1984; **288**: 1355–9.
3 MacLeod D. Sport and Exercise Medicine. Medio-legal issues and the doctor. *J Med Dent Def Union* 1997; **3**: 4–5.
4 Bolam *v*. Friern Hospital Management Committee. 1957; QBD BMLR 1,1.
5 MacLeod DAD. MacLeod's guidelines for doctors in sport. *Br J Sports Med* 1998; **32**: 48.
6 Day AT. Exercising medical judgement. *Br J Sports Med* 1997; **31**: 266.

17 The doctor on tour

Travelling with a team presents a particular challenge. There are three main phases to this responsibility. The pre-travel phase, the travel phase and the doctor on location. A major paper outlining the preparations for a major event such as the Commonwealth Games has been published [1]. Planning should begin well in advance, focusing on the players, the climate, time zone changes and immunisations. The size of the medical team is usually determined by the finance available but the players are the priority and there is always a trade-off between what is ideal and what can be financed. For a tour of any significance the minimum medical team is a doctor and a physiotherapist. Ideally the doctor, or at least some responsible member of management, should travel out beforehand to see the environment, the hotel and its facilities, and plan the diet. If the tour location is very hot, then they should also address the issue of fluid replacement. It is essential to inspect the medical facilities at the venue, access to hospitals and find out how to order prescriptions or medication. If the team is of reasonable size there should be an identifiable medical room. At the very least, the doctor should have a separate room with a couch and an examination area.

Players travelling to some of the more exotic locations may require immunisations and malaria prophylaxis. Clearly, it makes sense to prepare well in advance and to be immunised outside competition time. This is sometimes difficult as team selection may only be made at the last minute. Every athlete should have updated basic immunisations to diptheria, tetanus and polio. In more exotic locations, there may be health risk from malaria; also typhoid and hepatitis A and B are significant illnesses and may require prophylaxis. The athlete will also wish to avoid any possible morbidity or side-effects associated with immunisation so this should be undertaken well before travel to the event. If the immunisation schedule is complex or time is short, it is best to seek expert advice. Details of the immunisations appropriate for different countries are available both in MIMS and in the BNF, but specialist advice is available from the local travel clinic or from the Infectious Diseases Centre at Colindale. Needs of the athlete may vary depending on the sport. Cyclists and distance runners who may be training far from their accommodation may have more need of rabies vaccine than swimmers. Similarly a boxer is more likely to be exposed to hepatitis B than a gymnast. Sailors, canoeists and rowers may be more likely to be exposed to malaria than tennis players. In a multisport team, needs may vary if athletes are competing in one or more venues. Competitors may also plan a holiday after the event and they may require additional vaccinations or malaria prophylaxis. An individual may decide to forego some of the immunisations after discussion with his or her own general practitioners but the team doctor should give the appropriate general advice.

Malaria prophylaxis may also be recommended depending on the location. Anti-mosquito measures are just as important as medication and are often forgotten. Clothing and insect repellant should be used by day and anti-mosquito nets used by night. Athletes should be advised on treatment and use the appropriate prophylaxis according to the most recent guidance.

Travel to the venue

Time zone and heat acclimatisation are important factors for the travelling athlete. The time spent at a training camp or competition venue is often dictated by finance so that the athlete may not have sufficient time to acclimatise before competing. Heat acclimatisation depends on the individual and their response to temperature and humidity. If travelling to altitude there may be additional problems.

Travelling affects different athletes in different ways but may be a major factor in performance. In many cases athletes travel around the globe to competition venues crossing many time zones. The effects of jet lag can be considerable. Experienced athletes learn to cope with jet lag in their own way. Some take sleeping tablets, some take melatonin, some simply try to sleep through the journey. Sleeping tablets may be effective but some athletes find the sedative effect disconcerting and they have a prolonged period of sedation in spite of a short pharmacological half-life. There is evidence that benzodiazepines can impair concentration and reaction time even 12 hours afterwards. While this may not be a major problem if travel is some time before com-petition, they should clearly be avoided the night before a major event where reaction time and concentration are important. The effects of melatonin are not well researched but empirically many believe that it works. Melatonin is a naturally occurring hormone and peak levels usually occur at night where it has a key role in coordinating the body's physiological clock. In the-ory, taking melatonin can help reset the body clock and adjust to a new time zone. In practice the effects can be unpredictable. Melatonin is, as yet, not freely available in the UK and is not recommended by the British Olympic Association [2]. In-experienced athletes should not try either medication for the first time on their way to a major games. It is best to experiment away from the critical pre-event period. Sleeping on aeroplanes is difficult anyway and there is always great excitement when travelling to a major event. It is unlikely, therefore, that in-experienced air travellers will have any significant rest during the journey.

It is also very difficult for a fit athlete, used to a very active life, perhaps training 6 hours each day to adjust to the cramped space in an aeroplane seat for perhaps more than 12 hours. Athletes eat a lot, and the meals on the plane may be quite inadequate so additional food may be required. Air travel is also dehydrating so they should drink copiously during the flight. They should avoid alcohol as it has a diuretic effect adding to the dehydrating effect of air travel. Some athletes suffer motion sickness. They should think about this in advance and take appropriate medica-tion but should have tried this medication before travelling to a major event.

After a long journey crossing time zones, one thing is certain, the fit healthy athlete who left home in the best condition of a lifetime, will arrive at their destination feeling ghastly. The com-bined effects of excitement, inactivity, lack of sleep and arrival in a foreign country in a different climate and time zone take their toll. Some athletes may be unable to train properly for up to 1 week, depending on the venue and time of travel.

Time zone adaption is more difficult travelling from West to East. If the athlete is travelling from East to West, from Europe to North America for example, and will only be present for a short period, it may be useful to avoid time zone adaptation at all and try to maintain European time. If intending to adapt to the local time, athletes should begin to plan long before travelling. In the days before travelling, they should begin to alter their sleep pattern towards the destination night time hours, if only by one or two hours. When travelling, they should alter their watches as soon as the arrive on the plane. They should avoid alcohol when flying and try to sleep at the appropriate times. Sleep may be helped by taking one of the short acting hypnotic agents.

At the venue

There is a surprisingly high demand on medical services both at training camp and at competition. Doctors may wonder how such a bunch of fit healthy athletes at the peak of condition can at the same time be such hypochondriacs. The team doctor is on call for 24 hours each day from the moment the team assembles and will often have to respond to many simple and trivial problems at the most unpredictable moments. If allowed to develop, medical care can become a completely unstructured series of unsatisfactory bar room and bus stop consultations. In order to bring some structure it is usually best to set up organised surgery hours so that both athletes and doctors have some protected medical time together. Casual consultations always happen, of course, but at least there is a planned contact point where the athlete can be certain of a proper consultation. The planned consultation time should ideally coincide with breakfast and evening meal so that consultations occur early in the morning at a time when the doctor and physiotherapist can put together a treatment strategy, and the coach adjust the training plan. Confidentiality is essential, proper records should be maintained, and the player's own doctor should be kept informed.

Traveller's diarrhoea

Food acclimatisation is one of the factors least considered when a team travels abroad. Even with rigorous adherence to food preparation and hygiene, travellers are inevitably exposed to different flora in water and foodstuffs. Adjustment of the gut flora may give transient diarrhoea. Athletes, as other travellers, are most susceptible to gastrointestinal upset and diarrhoea when travelling to developing countries in particular. The term minor gastrointestinal upset is commonly used, but for the elite level athlete hoping to compete at their best, the term minor illness is a misnomer. Most travelling athletes have suffered from diarrhoea at some stage in their career. Traveller's diarrhoea is a big problem for the athlete who may be competing at a major event where performance is critical. Diarrhoea can harm performance both through the debilitating effect of the infection itself and the secondary effects of dehydration. Medications used to slow intestinal motility often have atropine-like effects, which although reducing diarrhoea symptoms, make competitive exercise uncomfortable. Traveller's diarrhoea is usually due to exposure to different food pathogens, the most common of which is E. Coli. This condition is self limiting but with symptoms of watery diarrhoea, abdominal cramps, nausea, vomiting and weakness, it is far from a minor illness. Salmonella, Shigella and Campylobacter can all cause similar symptoms. Those travelling abroad should be aware of the standard advice on food: avoid salads and seafood, eat only well-cooked food, peel all fruits, do not eat food purchased on the street (especially ice creams) drink only bottled water and avoid ice in drinks. If diarrhoea occurs, the treatment is symptomatic by ensuring adequate hydration though fluid replacement. Electrolyte drinks are appropriate. For those with very severe diarrhoea, diphenoxylate (Lomotil) or loperamide (Imodium) may be used. These medications do, of course, have some atropine-like effects and the athlete who attempts to compete will be exceptionally uncomfortable from the combined effects of dehydration and the atropine-like side-effects. Those with acute diarrhoea should be isolated from the remainder of the touring party and very strict hygiene measures initiated. Occasionally hospital admission for intravenous fluid replacement is required. Some athletes may wish to take prophylactic antibiotics. A suitable antibiotic regime would be trimethoprim 200 mg b.d. for 5 days or ciprofloxacin 500 mg b.d. which will also cover against Campylobacter.

Occasionally a major outbreak of diarrhoea can occur at a sporting event. This can have a catastrophic effect, such as occurred with a major outbreak at a world junior rowing championships [3]. At this event 10% (78) of all competitors had diarrhoea. There were 104 consultations in one national team and athletes were treated with Dioralyte rehydration solution, loperamide, cinnarizine, paracetamol and ciprofloxacin. A medical officer from another competing nation treated six athletes with intravenous fluid replacement in their rooms and five athletes from other teams required hospital admission.

Sun protection

Sun burn is a risk, even in temperate climates. We are increasingly aware of the risk of excessive sun and the adverse effects of ultra-violet light exposure. Ideal sun protection is provided by long sleeves, a hat and topical sun screens but athletes may have to be reminded about this. Those competing on the water, sailing, rowing and canoeing are at particular risk, and those with dark skin can burn too. Individuals should be aware of this and wear adequate protection but the team management should plan in advance and supply appropriate protection, both in kit and sun screens.

References

1 Young M, Fricker P, Maughan R, MacAuley D. The travelling athlete: issues relating to the Commonwealth Games, Malaysia, 1998. *Br J Sports Med* 1998; **32**: 77–81.
2 Policy Statement of the British Olympic Association. *Br J Sports Med* 1998; 1.
3 Anderson AC. Outbreak of salmonella food poisoning at Junior World Rowing Championships. *Br J Sports Med* 1996; **30**: 347–8.

18 Acclimatisation

Altitude

Travelling to altitude used to be considered an essential part of preparation for endurance sport by any serious athlete. In general practice one is more commonly asked about the effects of altitude by tourists travelling to South America or on walking holidays in Himalayas or the Alps. Those who have cardiorespiratory impairment should avoid such high altitude activity holidays with the added physiological stress of altitude. Paradoxically, those who are fittest often suffer most from altitude sickness. The early symptoms, which almost everyone experiences, include a dry mouth, poor sleeping and mild breathlessness. These symptoms may be exacerbated by the reduced humidity at altitude. More severe altitude or acute mountain sickness gives symptoms similar to acute cardiac failure with dyspnoea, pulmonary oedema and later cyanosis. The only effective treatment for acute mountain sickness is to return to a lower altitude. Some travel specialists recommend taking acetazolamide, a diuretic, which helps reduce acute mountain sickness. This subject is covered in more detail in a later section.

Acclimatisation to heat

Athletes living and training in temperate climates are at considerable disadvantage when competing in a hot and humid environment, even highly trained athletes. It is the combination of heat and high humidity which creates the greatest stress, hence the use of wet bulb globe temperature (WBGT) as the index of overall environmental heat stress [1]. Guidelines on prevention of heat-related injury have been published by the American College of Sports Medicine [2]. Those most affected are those competing in endurance sports where performance is inevitably impaired, but those playing field games may also be at risk when playing in mid-day temperatures. The ability to maintain body temperature is a key factor in athletic performance. Heat, or the inability to adapt, together with dehydration may greatly harm athletic performance. Heat and humidity should be considered together, because while heat acclimatisation is important it is considerably more difficult in conditions of high humidity. In high ambient temperatures the body stays cool mainly through evaporation and can maintain core temperature to within 3–4°C. In high humidity, heat loss through evaporation is not as effective.

The time required to acclimatise depends on the temperature and humidity. The body can adapt to heat in a number of ways. At first, the body is unable to cope with heat and players become fatigued and easily tired. Performance is impaired and the cardiovascular stress of exercise is greater [3]. As the player adapts the speed of onset, rate and distribution of sweating increase and the heart rate and exercise heart rate decrease. It takes 1–2 weeks to adjust to a warmer climate [4] and in the early period of adaptation the training sessions should be reduced in intensity and duration. These reduced sessions should continue for at least 1 week. All other factors remaining the same, exercise in the heat is a greater physiological load, reflected in a higher heart rate. It is important to exercise, however, to aid adaptation. Many athletes attempt to begin this adaptation before travelling abroad by training in a hot and humid environment either in their bathrooms or wearing layers of clothing and sweat tops. This may be effective [5]. With heat acclimatisation the main physiological changes that occur are an increase in blood volume and an increased ability to sweat. Sweating occurs earlier and in greater volume. With longer duration heat exposure, further adaptation occurs with a reduced sweat concentration and lower sodium content.

Organisation of travelling and training camp arrangements are the prerogative of the management and the time spent at the venue will be a balance of a number of factors, including finance, in team preparation. The medical team should try to influence management plans on the basis of the need for acclimatisation.

When preparing for an event the athlete should attempt to train at the same time as the competitive event in order to prepare for similar conditions, rather than train at a time when the temperature is least. On first arrival the athletes should not immediately attempt to train under race conditions but gradually expose themselves during light training, while doing their more intense work in the cooler part of the day. They may then gradually increase their time and heat exposure. Needless to say, those competing should wear suitable lightweight, and light in colour, clothing. Even with suitable preparation, and appropriate clothing and hydration, performance in endurance events will inevitably be affected.

Athletes should avoid lounging around in the heat, sun bathing should be prohibited and they should take full advantage of shade and air-conditioning. Those intending to travel to a major event in hot and humid conditions should, if at all possible, try to experience similar conditions beforehand in a training camp or at competition. It is unrealistic to expect athletes to get it right first time, and experience is a great teacher for those who doubt the importance of preparation and acclimatisation.

The two main problems associated with training and competing are dehydration and hyperthermia and while acclimatisation can help adapt to the conditions, these two potential problems always persist. Chronic dehydration occurs when the athlete trains in hot conditions but does not make up the fluid loss. This can easily occur where athletes do not appreciate the volume of fluid loss and are unaccustomed to drinking sufficient to make good such fluid deficit. Athletes should be aware of the huge potential fluid loss, and should also be aware that thirst is not a good index of fluid deficit and that they will need to make a particular effort to maintain fluid balance. There are a number of methods of gauging fluid loss. The simplest is through daily weighing, preferably in the morning before eating or drinking. The athlete should be able to compare their day-to-day weight fluctuation with their previous training and racing weight. Those competing at weight categories will be acutely aware of their body weight but others may not know their previous weight accurately. Monitoring fluid loss is especially important in weight category and endurance sports. Those competing in weight category sports may be tempted to use dehydration as a short cut to making the weight. This carries risk as there is a significant loss in quality of performance with dehydration. Even a 2% loss of body weight can result in a significant impairment [6]. Therefore, those competing in weight category sports should be encouraged to make the weight long before their competition. The medical officer should work closely with the athletes and management in such sports long before the competition. Experienced competitors will have their own weight loss strategy planned well in advance. Weight loss during each training session may also be recorded and as most of this is fluid loss this should serve as a preliminary daily target for fluid replacement. A second method is by monitoring the urine. This may be by simply observing the colour and ensuring that one drinks sufficient to pass clear colourless urine. A more objective method may be by monitoring the urine specific gravity.

The major problem is that dehydration can harm athletic performance. When competing in one's own locality, variations in environmental conditions may affect performance but the day-to-day variation is the same for all. Climatic adaptation becomes much more important at international level where athletes and teams may travel to major events in very different environments. Athletes and team managers should be able to anticipate these very different conditions and prepare appropriately.

Acute dehydration occurs when an athlete becomes dehydrated during a training session or event. This is closely linked with hyperthermia. The athlete becomes extremely hot but is unable to lose heat. They may become confused, irrational and collapse and acute heat illness is a serious medical emergency.

Profuse sweating may cause salt loss and those training and competing in conditions of very high temperature should take salt supplements. Hyperthermia is a particular problem in maximal exertion where the body cannot lose heat quickly enough. Adaptation can speed the process of heat loss, but hyperthermia can still occur.

Fluid replacement in a hot environment

Players should be encouraged to drink and contrary to what some athletes expect, fluid replacement becomes more important as the athlete becomes acclimatised and sweating becomes more efficient. Thirst is a very poor indication of dehydration and the quantity of fluid required depends on each individual's fluid loss. The athlete should try to estimate the expected fluid loss on a daily basis and plan to consume this quantity. The volumes required can be quite substantial and it may take the athlete some days to become accustomed to drinking such a volume of fluid. Some athletes find it difficult to consume large volumes of fluid during competition or training but in very hot conditions athletes should aim for a target intake of approximately 500 ml per hour. Clearly this will vary according to the athlete, the sport and the conditions, but athletes like to have a target and 500 ml is a reasonable estimate. If playing a field sport, fluid can be consumed before the match and at half time, but players should also make use of every other opportunity at every break in play. When in training, athletes should have fluid bottles with them at all times and drink constantly. Drinking should be for prevention of dehydration rather than treatment, and an athlete should aim never to become dehydrated. Ideally their fluid intake should be constant, drinking about 150 ml every 15 minutes. There are particular problems when sweat loss exceeds the theoretical maximum rate of gastric emptying and hence potential fluid absorption. Gastric emptying is also slowed by anxiety and by high intensity sport. Clearly there are problems in very hot climates where sweat loss of more than 1.5 litres per hour, exceeds the normal gastric emptying of about 1 litre per hour and dehydration seems almost inevitable. It is essential that athletes minimise the problems of dehydration by learning to drink large volumes and tolerate this intake while competing. In very severe climatic conditions, there have been reports of team doctors administering intravenous fluids during half time in some events.

Most athletes use proprietary sports drinks which contain carbohydrate and electrolytes. The optimum carbohydrate content varies according to the sport and balance of fluid and energy need. Most drinks contain 5–7% carbohydrate. Additional sodium replacement is generally not required unless the exercise is of very long duration, high intensity, with very large sweat loss. In most cases, some additional salt with one's food is sufficient. Some of the sodium deficit can be replaced using sports drinks which contain 10–25 mmol/l sodium. Sodium does have another important function, however, which is in maintaining thirst and a sports drink which quenches thirst before adequate fluid replacement is not effective. It is not easy for the athlete to drink large volumes of water and water ingestion alone may inhibit thirst. Maughan and colleagues [7] in their comprehensive review of rehydration, point out that a sweat loss of 5 litres with a sodium content of 50 mmol/l requires ingestion of 15 g of sodium chloride to restore balance. This magnitude of salt loss is not replaced in a normal diet. Clearly choosing a fluid replacement drink should reflect the environmental conditions and the expected sweat loss.

Preparing for competition in a hot environment

There are a number of key factors that determine the appropriate preparation for competition in a hot environment. Adaptation to heat occurs in 1–2 weeks but during this period the intensity of training must be reduced. Ideally one would attempt to speed up this adaptation in preparation for a major event. This may be through preparation at home or at a warm weather training camp. The method chosen will depend on the location of the event and the funding available. The sporting organisation should also try to ensure that an athlete's first exposure to heat is not in a major competition and that they have had the opportunity to experience the difficulties of training and racing in a hot environment prior to this major event.

Home preparation

For those who wish to adapt to the heat and humidity of a competition venue before an event there are two alternatives. The first is to travel to the competition site or a location with a similar climate for a training period beforehand. Alternatively one may attempt to undertake some climatic adaptation before travelling. Those hoping to acclimatise at home may train in a climatic chamber or try to produce their own heat stress by training heavily clothed or in wet weather suits [5]. The ideal preparation may be to combine both home preparation and location acclimatisation.

One may prepare by intermittent training in a hot environment. Exercising in the heat every third day for 30 days is as effective as every day for 10 days and sessions of about 60–100 minutes duration should be undertaken once or twice weekly. This may be introduced into the normal training programme without much major disruption. These sessions should be of sufficient intensity to raise core temperature and need not be continuous so they may be made up of a number of shorter more intense sessions. It may be difficult to find a suitable hot training space but the mode of training is not critical and any form of training that raises core temperature is satisfactory.

Training camp

The environmental conditions at training camp should mimic those of the event and coaches and managers should modify training to prepare for the event. It makes sense to balance training so all is not undertaken at the time of maximum heat and to alter the time of training so that there is a gradual introduction to maximum heat stress, but that there is still adequate heat exposure for adaptation. The time from arrival to return to maximum intensity training should be about 5 days. In these early days of heat adaptation the training load should be light in intensity and of short duration.

During training and competition the athlete should take every opportunity to stay in the shade and should maintain fluid intake. When not training or competing they should try to remain indoors in the cool air-conditioned environment. Temperature and humidity contribute to the heat stress and the method used to quantify the combined effect is the wet bulb globe temperature (WBGT). The formula used is

$$WBGT = 0.7[WB] + 0.2[GT] + 0.1[DB]$$

Where   WB = relative humidity-wet bulb,
              GT = black globe temperature,
              DB = dry bulb.

Further details of advice on coping with heat is to be found in the position stand of the American College of Sports Medicine [2].

References

1 Sparling PB. Expected environmental conditions for the 1996 summer Olympic games in Atlanta. *Clin J Sports Med* 1995; **5**: 220–2.
2 American College of Sports Medicine. Prevention of thermal injuries during distance running. *Med Sci Sports Exer* 1987; **19**: 529–33.
3 Galloway SDR, Maughan RJ. Effects of ambient temperature on the capacity to perform prolonged exercise in man. *J Physiol* 1995; **489**: 35–6.
4 Armstrong LE, Maresh CM. The induction and decay of heat acclimatisation in trained athletes. *Sports Med* 1991; **12**: 302–12.
5 Dawson B. Exercise training in sweat clothing in cool conditions to improve heat tolerance. *Sports Med* 1994; **17**: 233–44.
6 Armstrong LE, Costill DL, Fink WJ. Influence of diuretic-induced dehydration on competitive running performance *Med Sci Sports Exer* 1985; **17**: 456–61.
7 Maughan RJ, Leiper JB, Shirreffs SM. Factors influencing the restoration of fluid and electrolyte balance after exercise in the heat. *Br J Sports Med* 1997; **31**: 175–82.

19 Outdoor and mountain pursuits

Not just mountaineers climb mountains or go trekking at altitude. Many people now take vigorous outdoor holidays at altitude and travel to areas that would have only been visited by the very adventurous in the past. Often those who can afford to travel on these holidays are older and perhaps not as fit as they should be. They are likely to consult the general practitioner for medical advice and will expect a level of knowledge that may have been previously considered of a specialist nature. With modest ambitions and taking some reasonable precautions most people can safely enjoy a holiday at altitude.

Trekking and altitude sickness

Trekking in the Himalayas is no longer exotic, it is a package holiday accessible to many. It may be quite vigorous and require a basic level of fitness, although less ambitious expeditions are available. The main concern from a medical perspective is the effect of altitude and all the associated risks and hazards. With increasing altitude there is a decrease in atmospheric pressure, a reduction in alveolar oxygen tension and a reduction in oxygen saturation. At sea level the blood is 96% saturated but by 2,300 m (7,500 ft) oxygen saturation will have fallen below 90%. The proportion of oxygen in the air is the same but because there is less atmospheric pressure less oxygen is available. Up to 1,500 m (5,000 ft) there is little effect on oxygen saturation but, as a rule of thumb, oxygen saturation is reduced by about 10% with every 1,000 m. Problems usually begin above about 2,300 m (7,500 ft) and it is interesting to note, for comparison, that the Mexico Olympics were held at 2,240 m and that Everest is 8,848 m.

Almost everyone who travels to altitude experiences at least some symptoms. In most cases problems arise because people travel too quickly to altitude without allowing themselves the opportunity to acclimatise. Symptoms may include mild insomnia, headache, dry throat, lightheadedness, giddiness, poor sleeping, irritability, nausea and weakness. The short-term physiological effects are an increase in heart rate and respiration. This increase in respiration, which is the body's natural response in order to maintain oxygen saturation, is similar in effect to hyperventilation because it lowers CO_2 which in turn alters the acid–base balance. It is these metabolic changes which cause the adverse effects. Symptoms begin within 6–12 hours of arrival at altitude and may persist for 1–4 days. In most cases these symptoms resolve, but until they do, travellers should stop climbing, rest and wait for improvement. It is foolish to carry on regardless, whatever the time limitations, because symptoms may become more florid and life threatening.

The more serious manifestations of altitude sickness are acute pulmonary oedema, cerebral oedema and retinal haemorrhages. High altitude pulmonary oedema causes acute dyspnoea. While the signs and symptoms are very similar to the acute pulmonary oedema that occurs in congestive cardiac failure, the aetiology is different and diuretic therapy is of little benefit. In mild cases, dyspnoea may be slight, with a cough, tiredness and some congestive signs on auscultation. In mild cases the treatment is rest but in more severe cases, with acute dyspnoea, the only option is to return to lower altitude.

High altitude cerebral oedema causes severe headache, ataxia, altered mental status with psychological symptoms. Judgement can be affected so that important decisions about continuation of a holiday or climb must be made by others. Ultimately acute cerebral oedema may progress to loss of consciousness. This is a medical emergency. While the symptoms may be treated with oxygen and dexamethasone, the only definitive treatment is return to a lower altitude.

Retinal haemorrhages may occur at high altitude. They occur more commonly in climbers and those who are very active. Haemorrhages that affect vision, macular haemorrhages for example, are an ophthalmological emergency and the patient should return to lower altitude.

Altitude sickness occurs frequently and the incidence seems to be increasing, perhaps due to the ease and rapid travel to altitude without a gradual acclimatisation period. In mild cases the treatment may be symptomatic, but the patient must rest. In more severe cases the only definitive treatment is return to lower altitude. The key to prevention is a gradual ascent to altitude, which allows the traveller to acclimatise gradually. In the past when transport was much more difficult, this acclimatisation was an integral part of travel, but now with ease of flying and motorised transport, visitors can travel to altitude very rapidly.

When first arriving at high altitude, visitors should allow at least 24 hours to acclimatise before exercise. Simply living at altitude is a physiological stress but those who are fittest are usually those most anxious to get going, and paradoxically are often those most likely to suffer. At altitude, dehydration is also a problem compounded by the increased respiratory effort so adequate fluid replacement is a priority. Diet is important and a high carbohydrate diet is recommended. Those on holiday, or adjusting to jet lag, may be tempted to consider alcohol or night sedation, but this is contraindicated. Travellers must also guard against sunburn.

There are a number of methods used to help prevent acute mountain sickness [1]. The best method of preventing acute mountain sickness is a slow ascent. There is some evidence that acetazolamide may be an aid to prevention and many climbers take it prophylactically. The dose for adults is 250 mg twice daily, or as 500 mg in a slow release formulation, starting at least one day before travel. Also dexamethasone (4 mg q.d.s.) has been used both in prevention in the short term with a course no longer than 2–3 days and in treatment.

Experienced climbers experience altitude sickness too. Usually they are well aware of the risk and plan their travel to base camp and ascent accordingly. Climbers at very high altitude 'climb high and sleep low' and have very gradually staged ascents above 10,000 ft (3,000 m).

Hypothermia

Hypothermia occurs when core body temperature falls; core body temperature should be measured rectally. Clinical symptoms begin at about 35°C with shivering, poor coordination and there may be some impairment of mental function. Hypothermia is more likely to occur in cold, wet, windy conditions and when tired. It occurs even in temperate climates, when the combination of cold ambient temperature, rain and wind can rapidly cool the body. The effect of the wind can provoke considerably greater heat loss than would occur at the same temperature in still conditions. Wind chill factor is an estimate of this effect.

Body heat is maintained by muscular activity so that when an exercising athlete or hill walker gets tired or hungry and is unable to keep up sufficient muscle activity to generate body heat, their temperature falls quickly. If competing in an athletic event, where they may be dressed in minimal clothing, or in clothes designed specifically to aid heat loss, body temperature can fall rapidly when they slow down. Moderate hypothermia can occur, for example, in the untrained marathon runner who, dressed in a running vest and shorts with no protection against unexpected wind and rain, tires after 15 or 20 miles, slows down, and cannot generate heat. Similarly the cyclist who although wet, could maintain core body temperature by the heat generated from muscle activity in cycling, becomes cold very rapidly when they stop to mend a puncture.

The symptoms of hypothermia include poor speech, poor concentration and shivering. The more alarming symptoms are of impaired judgement and a feeling of 'don't care'. These symptoms, especially if occurring on a mountain walk or expedition may put at risk the lives of both the patient and his or her companions. To prevent hypothermia, proper clothing is the key. This should use several protective layers and avoidance of clothes that absorb and retain water. Walkers and climbers should not wear 'jeans'; these absorb water, retain water and dry slowly. A hat is essential as up to 10% of body heat may be lost from the head. Alcohol should not be used in treating hypothermia as it causes peripheral vasodilatation and encourages heat loss.

The appropriate treatment is by gradual warming. A sudden warming of the peripheries causes a sudden increase in venous return of very cold blood reducing core body temperature further.

Cold slows down metabolism and the unconscious casualty may survive much longer than expected. In cold conditions, especially after immersion in cold water, an apparently dead victim may in fact survive leading to the well-known advice to casualty officers 'it is not enough to be cold and dead, one must be warm and dead'.

Frostbite

Frostbite occurs when parts of the body are frozen. It is most common in distal parts of the body where heat loss is greatest such as the fingers, toes, ears and nose. There is local tissue damage and ischaemic damage may be permanent so that frost bite may lead to loss of digits. Prevention is the key through adequate clothing and activity. The early symptoms in frostbite are numbness. If this occurs in the feet this may lead to more serious traumatic damage if walking, for example, in a expedition. The appropriate treatment of frostbite is gradual warming but the greatest damage occurs in tissues that are thawed and then refrozen. With thawing of the tissue there may be extreme pain so analgesia is required.

Chilblains are a common general practice complaint for which there is no effective treatment. The key is prevention, as chilblains occur most often from cold.

References

1 Coote JH. Medicine and mechanisms in altitude sickness. Recommendations. *Sports Med* 1995; **20**: 148–59.

20 Exercise and illness

Exercise is important for the healthy, to help keep them healthy, but exercise can also be important for those with medical conditions. Patients may have a chronic illness or be physically impaired but they need not be disabled. There are many reasons to be active at least in some way. People with chronic illness, coronary artery disease for example, are encouraged to be active and exercise has a place in the management of many other chronic medical conditions.

Respiratory disease

Respiratory disease is not an exclusion to exercise and those with asthma and chronic obstructive pulmonary disease (COPD) can often exercise without any problem. There is a relationship between physical activity and lung function in the general population so that those who are most active tend to have better FVC (forced vital capacity) and FEV_1 (forced expiratory volume in 1 s). It is not clear if this is due to cause or effect, as those who are most active may have improved lung function because of their activity or conversely those with reduced lung function may be least active. There is, however, little evidence that exercise can help improve lung function. In population studies, after excluding those with severe lung impairment, there is little relationship between lung function and physical fitness. Any impairment of lung function is important, however, for athletes and those exercising at high intensity.

While those with grossly impaired lung function are least likely to be active, minor lung function impairment is unlikely to affect physical performance. At the top levels of performance, highly trained individuals often reach their mechanical limits of lung and respiratory muscle for producing alveolar ventilation [1], but the mechanical limits to pulmonary ventilation are not reached until VO_2max. The oxygen cost of ventilation demand at maximal exercise in athletes averages 13% of VO_2max [2]. If there was increased demand due to expiratory obstruction, in asthma for example, this would create a greater proportional load on VO_2max. Research exploring this field is limited but there is some evidence of a decline in exercise tolerance with decline in FEV_1 with a close relationship between exercise capacity and severity of airflow limitation. It is unlikely, however, that ventilation is a major limiting factor in exercise with the exception of highly trained athletes during exhaustive exercise [3].

Smoking

Although FEV_1 falls gradually over a lifetime, clinically significant airflow obstruction does not usually develop in most non-smokers and many smokers. In some smokers irreversible obstructive changes do occur [4] and smoking is, of course, a major factor in impairment of lung function. Smokers in general are less fit [5,6] and even young smokers (age 16–18 years) have lower endurance performance times [7]. This is true not just in cross-sectional studies where there is a difference in fitness between smokers and non-smokers, but even in cohort studies there is a greater decline in physical fitness and lung function in smokers after 7-year follow-up [8]. Smoking may also influence the response to training and where physical fitness of smokers and non-smokers is not significantly different at baseline, smokers improve less than non-smokers [9]. In this study, although smokers had significantly lower endurance performance times on fitness testing, their VO_2max values were not significantly different.

An interesting anomaly has been shown in some fitness tests where, although smokers had a shorter exercise time in a symptom limited treadmill exercise test, they had a longer duration to submaximal heart rate [10]. This has important implications for interpretation of fitness tests because this later achievement of submaximal heart rate may lead to overestimation of fitness among smokers.

Asthma

Asthma is one of the chronic medical conditions usually managed in general practice. The reversible airways obstruction that is asthma, may occur as a reaction to allergens, but it may also occur in response to exercise so that physical activity may provoke airways obstruction in susceptible individuals. All those with asthma react to exercise and even some who do not have overt asthma experience some wheezing on exercise. Bronchospasm may be provoked by changes in humidity associated with rapid respiration during exercise or due to changes in air temperature so that exercise-induced bronchospasm (EIB) is more common during the winter months. While moderate airways obstruction may be tolerable in a sedentary individual, minor respiratory impairment can be of major consequence to a top athlete. The peak flow meter may not be sufficiently sensitive to detect minor degrees of respiratory impairment and the diagnosis may be based on symptoms alone. If the EIB is severe, the athlete may describe a wheeze on exercise, especially in cold weather, but more commonly athletes describe an exercise induced cough. This is an irritating cough after severe exertion which may not be associated with a wheeze. These symptoms warrant treatment with the usual asthma medication. The commonly prescribed preventive and therapeutic agents taken by inhalation are appropriate but those dealing with competitive athletes liable to be drug tested must be familiar with the regulations regarding medications permitted in the individual's sport. If asthma is a chronic medical condition needing medication then a normal treatment protocol is appropriate. If, however, bronchospasm is simply an exercise-induced phenomenon then medication is most useful just before and at the time of exercise; β_2-agonists should be inhaled about 1 hour before the event and again within 10 minutes of the actual event. They may also be required afterwards.

The clinical implications of research findings are that we should encourage those with asthma to be physically active. There is good reason to believe, although admittedly the evidence is not strong, that participation will improve lung function. Good control is important and athletes should monitor lung function using a peak flow meter. This may not detect the changes in lung function or airways obstruction that occur in mild asthma and which occur most often when an athlete is training or competing in cold weather. Change in temperature and humidity stimulates histamine release and thus bronchospasm, so exercise-induced asthma occurs in those who exercise at a moderate to high intensity such as runners, cyclists or rowers especially when training or competing during cold weather. Exercise-induced bronchospasm may also occur in those sports which require bursts of high intensity exercise during cold weather. It is much less likely in a warm moist environment, so swimming is recommended. In preparation for exercise in cold weather, or when they expect the intensity of exercise to cause bronchospasm, athletes should use their inhalers at least 30 minutes before training or competing. They should use a preventive inhaler regularly. If in doubt check the inhalers permitted under IOC regulations.

Athletes may manipulate the physiological changes associated with asthma by taking advantage of the physiological postexercise refractory period. Exercise stimulates bronchospasm at first but this eases immediately after exercise with a short period of improvement. This refractory period after exertion may last for up to 2 hours. In order to minimise the effects of asthma on performance in competition the athlete can modify their warm-up so that, rather than using a short warm-up immediately before an event, the athlete can perform a prolonged intermittent preparation. This means a longer and more protracted warm-up with periods of exercise mixed with periods of rest but the aim is that competition occurs during the refractory period. The warm-up work-load may be the same as other competitors but it begins much earlier and is intermittent.

Exercise-induced asthma occurs in up to 15% of the population, and has a similar prevalence in athletes even at the highest level. While some asthmatics recognise the symptom pattern associated with exercise others assume that wheezing with exercise is normal. Exercise related cough is a common complaint so that athletes complain of a severe wheezy cough in the first 30 minutes after intense exercise which persists in a mild form for some hours. This is the result of bronchospasm induced by the severe exercise. The diagnosis of EIB may be made on history alone but can be confirmed using an exercise test. To do this, ask the athlete undertake an intense period of exercise and measure peak flow before and after each 10 minutes for about 30 minutes. Some authors suggest that a 10% decrease in peak expiratory flow rate (PEFR) is diagnostic, but 10% decrease would have a major impact on performance in an athlete and a reduction of less than 10% is often treated.

A further important feature of asthma is the diurnal variation and PEFR is usually lowest in the morning. This can be important for those athletes who are competing in events which have early morning heats or preliminary rounds. It is important, therefore, to try to plan well in advance.

Osteoarthritis

Many patients ask if long-term sport can cause arthritis. In osteoarthritis the cycle of deterioration and regeneration of cartilage that occurs in a normal joint is impaired. There are areas of cartilage damage which expose the underlying bone. There are changes in the surface of the joint, formation of cysts, osteophytes and later there may be an effusion and synovitis. There may be a hereditary component in some people but excess weight or previous joint damage are the main predictors. Osteoarthritis is, of course, incurable and our treatment is aimed at reducing pain and inflammation while maintaining mobility.

Most studies of the relationship between osteoarthritis and sport have been retrospective and their findings depend both on the nature of the sport and if there was any previous joint damage directly attributable to the sport itself. If joint damage had been sustained during a playing career, then it is much more likely that this damage will progress in the long term. Studies to support this conclusion, being retrospective, are subject to all the potential bias associated with this type of study. The early studies were mainly surveys of athletes and the results were inconclusive. Other better quality studies have shown a 2–4 fold increase in risk [11,12].

In one study there was an increase in prevalence of osteoarthritis in former soccer players, which may have been anticipated bearing in mind the nature of the sport and potential injury, but there was also an increase among ex-weightlifters. In a study of runners and tennis players, where articular damage is less likely, the ex-athletes had greater rates of radiologically diagnosed osteoarthritis [13]. After adjustment for height and weight the association was stronger and the study concluded that there was increased risk of radiological osteoarthritis in ex-athletes. Another study of long-time middle-aged runners found the same degree of osteoarthritis in the knees, spine and hands as non-runners but that they were less disabled, probably because of better aerobic fitness and muscular skeletal strength. Overall there appears to be an increased risk of osteoarthritis, especially of the hip and knee, associated with long duration sports activity.

Patients with established osteoarthritis have a different perspective. They are concerned that by undertaking physical activity they may exacerbate their condition. Exercise has, however, been shown to improve osteoarthritis in some studies. In one study, patients had improved function and less pain after a programme of walking [14]. Conditioning exercises which improve the strength of the quadriceps also reduce symptoms [15]. A recent randomised controlled trial [16] also showed that older disabled persons with osteoarthritis of the knee had modest improvements in measures of disability, physical performance and pain from participating in either an aerobic or a resistance exercise programme. The authors believed that these data suggested that exercise should be prescribed as part of the treatment for knee osteoarthritis. In general, exercise should be within the limits of the patient's pain and discomfort and appropriate for the joint affected. Swimming, which is a non-weight-bearing conditioning and aerobic exercise, is appropriate for most patients with osteoarthritis, particularly of the back, but is not suitable for those with arthritis of the cervical spine. Cycling is also an ideal exercise, except for those with arthritis in the patellofemoral joint.

Diabetes

An Indian physician named Suchruta first suggested exercise as a treatment in 600 BC but the hypoglycaemic effect of exercise was not demonstrated until 1919 by Allen. Most of the benefits from exercise are in managing type 2 diabetes but those with type 1 can also benefit, not just from the effect on blood glucose but also from the beneficial effect on hypertension and lipid profile [17].

There are two important features of the relationship between diabetes and exercise. First, exercise can help in the prevention of non-insulin-dependent diabetes and in balancing glucose control. Second, it is important to recognise the difficulties that diabetics may experience in matching glucose control with bouts of exercise. For the travelling athlete in particular it is important to monitor insulin and glucose levels, especially crossing multiple major time zones where dietary care and meal planning is essential.

Physical activity is important in the primary prevention of non-insulin-dependent diabetes mellitus [18] and there is considerable evidence that those who are physically active are at less risk of developing type 2 or adult-onset diabetes [19]. There is evidence that physical activity equivalent to 5.5 metabolic units (METS) or greater for 40 minutes or more per week is enough to gain a protective effect, even after controlling for possible confounding factors such as age, baseline fasting blood glucose, BMI, serum triglyceride, systolic blood pressure, family history and alcohol consumption [20]. One of the striking aspects of this study was that the protective effect of this moderate level of exercise was greatest in the group at highest risk who reduced their risk by over two thirds (64%). This is very strong supporting evidence that we should encourage those in the highest risk groups to undertake moderate physical activity (such activity would include brisk walking at 5 m.p.h. or more, gentle swimming, leisure cycling, tennis, basketball and aerobics).

There are few contraindications to participation in sport in well-controlled diabetes. By monitoring blood glucose and proper adjustment of insulin and calorie intake the diabetic athlete can take part in almost any activity [21]. Ideally there should be collaboration between the athlete, coach and physician in planning training and competition and specialised dietary advice may be required. The benefits for the diabetic patient in taking exercise are that it helps maintain body weight, reduces the incidence of hypertension and helps lower lipid levels which in turn reduces the risk of cardiovascular disease. Not least are the psychological benefits associated with participating in sport and living life to the full while managing a chronic disease.

The additional metabolic load of endurance sport may add to the difficulties in control. For more prolonged exercise the insulin dose may be reduced but for shorter less frequent exercise, it may be sufficient to supplement with carbohydrate. Endurance exercise for 30–35 minutes can be undertaken without problems, but if exercising for longer periods the athlete may encounter difficulties due to reduced glycogen stores in the liver and skeletal muscle. The exercise response is also altered. In those with normal glucose metabolism, there is a reduction in insulin with exercise and a corresponding increase in glucagon and epinephrine which helps hepatic glucose production. In type 1 diabetes there is no reduction in plasma insulin and insulin may indeed rise if the exercise is shortly after injection or due to an increase in the blood supply to the injection. The glucose response is not present which may lead to hypoglycemia. The diabetic athlete may also be more susceptible to hypoglycemia 6–12 hours after exercise. In contrast, exercise can increase insulin sensitivity and improve control in type 2 diabetics who may need to reduce their medication.

Diving is the one sport for which insulin-dependent diabetes is a contraindication. This is mainly because of the risk that unconsciousness may be missed, which is an additional risk to the diver and his or her buddy. Diabetic people should also be extremely alert to the risks in many adventure sports, such as rock climbing, pot holing etc. where immediate medical aid is not always at hand and where companions could be put at risk. Diabetics also need to take care in sports which are intermittent and of unpredictable duration and where the metabolic load is difficult to predict.

Resistance training is of value in improving blood lipid profiles, increased left ventricular wall contractability, decreased blood pressure, improved insulin sensitivity and glucose tolerance and increased bone and connective tissue strength. Strength training is appropriate except where there is proliferative retinopathy. Routine diabetic care is particularly important in the diabetic athlete, to exclude retinopathy before high intensity exercise and to be aware of the hazards of neuropathy and care of the feet. The diabetic athlete should always wear a medic alert tag, and inform friends and colleagues who should have access to glucagon.

There is little evidence that exercise reduces the long-term complications of type 1 diabetes. The Pittsburgh IDDM morbidity study, in long-term follow-up found no decrease in retinopathy through participation in team school sports but there was a suggestion of a reduction in cardiovascular disease and overall mortality. They concluded that activity may be associated with a reduced risk of microvasular complications and mortality in males [22].

Epilepsy

Epilepsy is not a contraindication to exercise and there is little evidence that epilepsy medication should affect physical performance. There are, however, some risks associated with exercise in poorly controlled epileptics and common sense should prevail in advising patients on suitable sport. Those with epilepsy must not dive. They are a risk both to themselves and their buddy. If they have an epileptic fit under water they will die, and their buddy may be put at risk too.

Migraine

Some patients report an increase in migraine associated with exercise. In these patients it is useful to prescribe prophylactic medication. Exercise-related headache is not unusual and responds to simple medication. 'Ice cream headache' can occur with sudden immersion in cold water, as in diving or surfing [23].

Viral infections

Upper respiratory tract infections can be a major problem for the serious athlete. Sporting patients are vulnerable to infection too and there is some suggestion of immunological impairment in those who are training excessively, which may put them at particular risk. The most common viral infections are the adenoviruses, enteroviruses (echo viruses) and the influenza viruses. There is a potential risk of myocarditis in viral illness, with coxsackie virus in particular, so athletes should be discouraged from training if suffering from a significant viral illness.

Viral infections are easily transmitted and can harm performance if an athlete is ill at a major event, ruining many years of meticulous preparation. There is no simple answer in prevention and treatment is symptomatic. Travelling abroad exposes athletes to additional risk of infection through the closed air circulation and confined space of an aeroplane, and the cramped conditions usually found in the athlete's accommodation or hotel. Antibiotics are often used empirically as there are few facilities available for rapid diagnosis of viral infection. An athlete with a viral infection should not train or race until fully recovered and certainly should not train or race when suffering from myalgia, tachycardia or pyrexia.

A number of common viral infections can be associated with loss of form or chronic fatigue in athletes. Following severe viral infections, including influenza and infectious mononucleosis, there is tiredness and it may take some days before a full return to training. Sometimes this period can be prolonged with an extended run of poor performance or loss of form and occasionally these symptoms can last as long as 6 months, which is the threshold for a formal diagnosis of chronic fatigue syndrome. Viral illnesses are one possible cause of loss of form, but the patient should be investigated to exclude other possible causes such as blood dyscrasias, and metabolic conditions such as diabetes and thyroid disease.

Athletes tend to feel that they are more susceptible to viral infections. Recent evidence suggests that they may be right and that there may be some impairment of the immune system in those who are most active. Nieman [24] suggests that the relationship between exercise and upper respiratory tract infections be modelled on the J-shaped curve. Moderate exercise can decrease the risk of URTI through positive changes in the immune system, but excess exercise may lead to depression of the immune system and elevation of epinephrine and cortisol. Although there is no overall clear pattern, recent research reveals a number of interesting findings. Moderate exercise appears to cause a leucocytosis and increase the lymphocyte count, especially T-cells. High intensity activity can reduce the level of T lymphocytes and natural killer cells for almost 24 hours, which may indeed reduce resistance to viral illness. Similarly intense exercise may also reduce the level of salivary antibodies (IgA and IgM). Other studies have pointed out the lower white cell count that occurs in some marathon runners and related this to viral infection, while glutamine (an amino acid essential for lymphocyte metabolism) is depleted after intense exercise. These findings may help us understand a little more about the relationship between exercise and the immune system and enable us to learn more about post viral fatigue and loss of form in athletes. There are wider implications and it has also been suggested that sustained intense exercise may, through its influence on the immune system, increase susceptibility to certain cancers, although there is no clear evidence as yet.

Infectious mononucleosis (glandular fever)

Infectious mononucleosis is a viral infection due to the Epstein Barr virus. It is common in young people and is one of the viral illnesses frequently blamed for loss of form in the athlete. This condition can be very frustrating as the only realistic treatment is rest. The usual presenting symptom is a sore throat, but athletes may present with loss of form with the condition being diagnosed on investigation. They may present with a rash, in particular following a reaction to ampicillin. There is often generalised lymphadenopathy and sometimes splenomegaly. Physicians should look for splenomegaly on clinical examination before allowing a recovering athlete back to sport, especially contact sport. Those who have a serological diagnosis of glandular fever should not train until splenomegaly has been excluded by abdominal ultrasound [25] because of the risk of rupture.

The diagnosis is usually confirmed using the Monospot test and a differential white cell count will show atypical lymphocytes. As most general practitioners will know, the test may be negative in the early stages and if the diagnosis seems likely clinically it is useful to repeat it in 2 weeks.

The athlete with glandular fever should rest for at least 6–8 weeks and when clinically well may increase their activity level very gradually, easing off again with any excessive tiredness. Most athletes are keen to get back to their previous level of activity and it is important to emphasis a graded return. This is the key to prevention of relapse.

Loss of form

Chronic fatigue syndrome has become more common in the general population and one may have expected that the sporting population, being predominantly young and fit would escape. Chronic fatigue syndrome may affect athletes who present with sustained loss of form. Overtraining and post viral fatigue are often blamed for unexpected loss of form but the symptoms of overtraining also mimic very closely the symptoms of depression. The links between psychological stress, impaired immunity, susceptibility to infection and overtraining have yet to be fully explored. Undoubtedly athletes can suffer a period of poor performance in training and competition after a significant viral illness. Systemic manifestations have been demonstrated such as persistent raised antibody titres and abnormal muscle enzyme levels and biopsy findings. There is as yet no conclusive evidence to point to a single cause or an effective treatment. At present the advice is to exclude other illness and treat symptomatically. A proportion will return to sport but a significant percentage retire from sport never having been able to return to their previous level of performance.

Other infections

Toxoplasmosis gondii is a zoonosis which can mimic the symptoms of infectious mononucleosis and has been implicated in loss of form. It is a protozoal infection which may be acquired from the faeces of animals. Infection may be transmitted from a pet dog or cat, but the athlete is also at risk from pets fouling training grounds and football pitches. The diagnosis is by serology and management is similar to infectious mononucleosis although the illness is usually of shorter duration.

Toxicara canis is a common infestation of the gastrointestinal tract in dogs which can be transmitted through faeces. When ingested by man it may infect the host causing allergic-type symptoms, asthma and splenomegaly. Blood tests may reveal eosinophilia. It is also a potential cause of blindness. The sporting link is through possible infestation during sport. Dog lovers should be prohibited from exercising their pets on playing fields where they may defaecate and are a hazard to those using the grounds.

Hepatitis A is a common infection in young adults. It is spread by the oral–faecal route and outbreaks can occur in groups of individuals living in close contact in a team or training camp. The symptoms are well known and include nausea, vomiting, fatigue, jaundice, anorexia and abdominal pain. Viral titres (IgM) will indicate current infection while IgG antibodies indicate previous infection. Liver function test will also be abnormal. The athlete should not be physically active until the symptoms and signs have return to normal. Those who are close contacts, in a team or training camp for example, may be given immunoglobin and those who are travelling abroad should be immunised before travel.

Hepatitis B is spread through sexual intercourse and infected blood products including shared needles. Systemic use of performance enhancing drugs does occur, but athletes who are tempted should be aware of the risks and hazards of sharing medication and equipment. Combat sports players should consider immunisation against hepatitis B because of the risk of infection from cuts and bleeding.

Sports players are not immune from HIV and indeed the disclosure that world-renowned athletes suffered from HIV infection should alert us all to the risk [26]. HIV infection is a potential risk in sport, a factor highlighted in recent guidelines from FIMS [27]. At present one can only advise governing bodies on the appropriate management of open wounds and bleeding during contact and combat sport. Those who sustain a wound should ensure that they are managed in an appropriate manner with sterile dressing etc. The greatest risk remains from sexual intercourse and shared needles.

Walkers, hikers and orienteers are exposed to other hazards closer to home. Ticks, which are common even in European countries, may carry disease. Ticks attach themselves to the skin and often go unnoticed for some time. They should be removed, but this requires some dexterity to remove the tick without leaving part of it behind or allowing it to inject the skin. Tick-borne diseases include Lyme disease which is increasingly recognised in the United Kingdom and tick-borne encephalitis.

Prevention of infection

Prevention is as important to athletes as to the normal population although clearly even a minor infection can have very serious implications for the athlete at the peak of condition preparing for a major event. It is difficult to avoid exposure to viral respiratory infections in normal daily life. Athletes may be even more susceptible to infection because they often live and train in close contact and in cramped conditions, travelling abroad, and training at the limits of endurance. They should take simple precautions such as not sharing water bottles, care in cooking and avoiding sexually transmitted disease. They should ensure they have had the immunisations appropriate for travel. Those with the early symptoms of infection should rest from training to allow the body's natural defence mechanisms to work most effectively.

Anorexia

Many athletes, both men and women, have eating disorders. There is considerable pressure on those competing in weight category sports to make the weight. Growing athletes fight a losing battle and as their weight creeps up they may be tempted to try short cuts by using diuretics or laxatives. Others abuse thyroxine. For those planning to compete at weight categories, weight loss or at least weight restriction is normal behaviour. But this is also combined with intense exercise. Weight restriction can become excessive and obsessive, and lead to minor or major psychological problems. In endurance sports, particularly long distance running, there is also a considerable advantage in low body weight which improves an athlete's aerobic power-to-weight ratio. Excessive emphasis can, however, lead to obsessive eating behaviour.

It is understandable, too, how some athletes are attracted by the exaggerated claims of particular diets or food supplements which allegedly give that extra edge to performance. As a result some eat a faddy or at least very unusual diet. Access to a dietician is important. Most top athletes have such access and it is always useful to encourage them to seek appropriate dietary advice.

Exercise and depression

There is a body of evidence showing the relationship between exercise and well-being. This is mirrored by research into the relationship between exercise and depression. Cross-sectional data show that those who exercise are less depressed and those with depression are less likely to be active. However, it is difficult to tease out if this relationship is due to cause or effect. Evidence from prospective trials is mixed and the only evidence showing a dose–response curve is that of Paffenbarger in 1994 who showed that relative risk was less in those who had greatest physical activity calorie utilisation. Other theories linking exercise and well-being suggest that mood improvements with exercise are due to endorphins, temperature or biochemical changes.

In one randomised controlled trial of volunteers undertaking a training programme there was in increase in fitness but no change in depression. There was an improvement in well-being in both groups! Looking at the overall pattern of research evidence, some exercise increases well-being but not fitness and some improves fitness but not well-being. The research evidence is taken mostly from those very mildly depressed but there appears to be little effect in normal people. One of the major problems is in defining the two variables, depression and physical activity.

There is also behaviour-type evidence that excessive exercise can lead to depressive type symptoms and that those who are training hard are more susceptible to depression. Some believe that constant stress leads to a decrease in neurotransmitters. This can be seen in changes in response to the POMS questionnaire where the athlete usually demonstrates an iceberg effect but with excessive exercise they show an inverted iceberg effect. While exercise is generally associated with a reduction in depression in those mildly depressed, excessive exercise may lead to depression in some individuals.

Exercise, cancer and the immune system

There is increasing interest in relationships between exercise and the immune system and emerging evidence for the protective effect of physical activity in relation to cancer. This evidence was first detected in relation to colon cancer but recent evidence also points to the protective effect in breast cancer and some weak evidence with prostate cancer.

The incidence of breast cancer is lower in women who exercise regularly [28]. In a study of over 25,000 women the risk was lower, by about 60%, after adjustment for age and body mass index, in those with greater leisure time physical activity. The risk reduction was greater in premenopausal women than in postmenopausal women who exercised regularly. This pattern was seen especially in those women under 45 years of age who exercised for at least 4 hours each week.

The exact model for the protective effect of moderate exercise against cancer is not known but it is suggested that cells of the monocyte-macrophage type may inhibit tumour growth and destroy cancer cells [29]. This is one potential beneficial effect of exercise on the host response to cancer. This research is at a very early stage and although the findings are encouraging, one cannot draw any firm conclusions. It is not known either if exercise can have any effect on established cancer. Cancer is not just one disease, but a variety of different conditions, and one cannot be sure that each tumour will react in the same manner.

There is evidence of a protective effect from moderate exercise on infection but also evidence that those who exercise excessively may be more susceptible [30]. This effect may be at cellular level. Acute bouts of exercise cause changes in the circulating mononuclear cells. There is an increase in lymphocyte count and alterations in natural killer cells, B cells and T cells. With chronic exercise the effect is opposite, the number of lymphocytes falls with impairment of their function and the duration of this effect depends on the exercise load. During this time cell-mediated immunity is impaired and the athlete is susceptible to infection [31]. In animal models physical activity increases the activity of killer T cells. This is still an emerging field and it is fascinating to compare the quantity of literature relating to cancer to that relating to cardiovascular disease. It is likely that this story will evolve as the evidence unfolds.

Diarrhoea in runners

Many runners suffer diarrhoea on running long distances. There are many possible causes. Some runners have intestinal hurry so that the bowel quickens on exercise, they were comfortable before they went out running but after about 30 minutes they feel the need to defaecate. This may be a purely physiological occurrence unrelated to food or drink but in others it is a result of nonabsorption of ingested fluid. High concentration drinks may, through their osmolality, draw fluid into the gut and diarrhoea results.

Blood loss can occur in faeces. Clearly faecal occult blood is an alarming symptom which requires investigation. One possible cause, having excluded more sinister aetiology, is the microscopic blood loss that may occur in runners. This may be due to intra-abdominal trauma causing 'caecal slap'.

Traveller's diarrhoea

If diarrhoea occurs, the athlete should rest completely, drink appropriate electrolyte fluids to avoid dehydration, and take an antidiarrhoea preparation such as Imodium or Lomotil. These medications have side-effects. The athlete should be isolated from other members of the squad to avoid infecting every one. Strict hygiene measures should be in place.

Prevention is most important. In most cases the symptoms are due to a change in gut flora rather than an overt infestation. Preventive measures are to ensure minimal exposure to infection. When travelling to many countries athletes should avoid all uncooked food, especially from street vendors, including salads, ice creams and ice cubes in drinks. Fruit should be peeled, and shellfish avoided. Some advocate taking antibiotics to prevent infection.

Exercise-induced urticaria

Some individuals are highly histamine sensitive and develop an exercise-induced itch or urticarial reaction on moderate exercise. This is the classical urticarial reaction with skin itch, red rash and raised red patches. Exercise-induced urticaria is a difficult problem and may be seasonal, more often occurring in the summer months. Treatment is by antihistamines but these may have a sedative effect and the decision to use them should be a joint decision between the athlete and the doctor taking into consideration the demands of the sport. The dose should be the minimum dose to control the symptoms.

Such urticarial symptoms may also occur in the athlete un-related to exercise. For example, some suffer from cold urticaria, others are very sensitive to water pressure in the shower or react if they take aspirin or non-steroidal anti-inflamatories for musculoskeletal problems.

Allergic rhinitis

This is characterised by a blocked runny nose with itching and general upper respiratory congestion and can cause considerable discomfort to an athlete. Pollen-induced allergies occur in the summer months and are typically associated with field sports. Allergic rhinitis can be a particular problem in cyclists. Individuals may be sensitive to particular pollens and their symptoms reflect the seasonal variation in pollen exposure, but some have a widespread and generalised sensitivity. Treatment is by both topical and oral medication. Athletes should be very careful about the use of medication as many preparations, including those bought over the counter without a prescription, contain pseudoephedrine and related compounds which are banned drugs under IOC regulations. Team doctors must emphasise that athletes should not use these preparations and in particular should not purchase 'over the counter' in other countries. Reading the label is no safeguard as not all constituents may be included and the names may not correspond directly to the list given in the IOC regulations. The IOC list is deliberately broad and includes the phrase 'and related compounds' so it is insufficient defence to say that the contents were not included on the banned list. Furthermore, the regulations on medicine listing in other countries may not require that all constituents be listed or the names of constituents may not be easily recognisable and the regulations covering 'health products' as opposed to medicines can be rather different.

Obesity

Evidence from public health studies suggests that obesity, at population level, is due to an imbalance of physical activity and calorie intake. Examining national statistics, there is a overall decrease in food consumption but an increase in the prevalence of obesity. The implication is that the increasing levels of obesity are due to an imbalance caused by physical inactivity. Obesity is a risk factor for many conditions, abdominal obesity in particular. It is possible to track obesity from childhood into adulthood and physical inactivity is the common factor.

References

1 Johnson BD, Saupe KW, Dempsey JA. Mechanical constraints on exercise hyperpnea in endurance athletes. *J Appl Physiol* 1992; **73**: 874–86.

2 Clark JM, Sinclair RE, Lenox JB. Chemical and non-chemical components of ventilation during hypercapnic exercise in man. *J Appl Physiol* 1980; **48**: 1065–76.

3 Dempsey JA. Is the lung built for exercise? *Med Sci Sports Exer* 1986; **18**: 1443–55.

4 Fletcher C, Peto R. The natural history of chronic airflow obstruction. *BMJ* 1977; **1**: 1645–8.

5 Conway TL, Cronan TA. Smoking, exercise and physical fitness. *Prev Med* 1992; **21**: 723–34.

6 Leon AS, Jacobs DR, Debacker G, Taylor HL. Relationship of physical characteristics and life habits to treadmill exercise capacity. *Am J Epidemiol* 1991; **133**: 1231–45.

7 Dressendorfer RH, Amsterdam EA, Odland TM. Adolescent smoking and its effect on aerobic exercise tolerance. *Phys Sportsmed* 1983; **11**: 108–19.

8 Sandvik L, Erikssen G, Thaulow E. Long term effects of smoking on physical fitness and lung function: a longitudinal study of 1393 middle aged Norwegian men for seven years. *BMJ* 1995; **311**: 715–18.

9 Hoad NA, Clay DN. Smoking impairs the response to a physical training regime: A study of officer cadets. *J R Army Med Corps* 1992; **138**: 115–17.

10 Sidney S, Sternfield B, Gidding SS *et al*. Cigarette smoking and submaximal exercise test duration in a biracial population of young adults: the CARDIA study. *Med Sci Sports Exer* 1993; **25**: 911–16.

11 Kujala UM, Kaprio J, Sarna S. Osteoarthritis of weight bearing joints of lower limbs in former elite male athletes. *BMJ* 1994; **308**: 231–4.

12 Vingard E, Alfredson L, Goldie I, Hogstedt C. Sports and osteoarthritis of the hip: an epidemiologic study. *Am J Sports Med* 1993; **21**: 195–200.

13 Spector T, Harris P, Hart DJ *et al*. Risk of osteoarthritis associated with long term weight bearing sports. *Arth Rheum* 1996; **39**: 988–95.

14 Petersen MGE, Kovar-Toledano PA, Otis JC *et al*. Effect of a walking programme on gait characteristics in patients with osteoarthritis. *Arthritis Care Res* 1993; **6**: 11–16.

15 Puett DW, Griffin MR. Published trials of non-medicinal and non-invasive therapies for hip and knee osteoarthritis. *Ann Intern Med* 1994; **121**: 133–40.

16 Ettinger WH Jr, Burns R, Messier SP *et al*. A randomized trial comparing aerobic exercise and resistance exercise with a health education program in older adults with knee osteoarthritis. The Fitness Arthritis and Seniors Trial (FAST) *JAMA* 1997; **277**: 25–31.

17 Hough DO. Diabetes mellitus in sports. *Med Clin N Am* 1994; **78**: 423–37.

18 Yki-Jarvinen H. Pathogenesisi of non-insulin dependent diabetes mellitus. *Lancet* 1994; **343**: 91–5.

19 Kriska AM, Blair SN, Pereira MA. The potential role of physical activity in the prevention of non-insulin dependent diabetes mellitus. In *Exercise and Sports Science Reviews* (Holloszy JO, Ed), Williams and Wilkins, Baltimore, MD 1994: 121–43.
20 Lynch J, Helmrich SP, Lakka T *et al*. Moderately intense physical activities and high levels of cardiorespiratory fitness reduce the risk of non-insulin dependent diabetes mellitus in middle aged men. *Arch Intern Med* 1996; **156**: 1307–14.
21 LaPorte RE, Dorman JS, Tajima N *et al*. Pittsburgh Insulin Dependent Diabetes Mellitus Morbidity and Mortality Study: Physical activity and diabetic complications. *Paediatrics* 1986; **78**: 6.
22 Harries M. Ice cream headache occurred during surfing in winter. *BMJ* 1997; **7108**: 609.
23 Nieman DC. Exercise, upper respiratory tract infection and the immune system. *Med Sci Sports Exer* 1994; **26**: 128–39.
24 Young M. What athletes often ask. Should I train when I have a cold and if not when can I return? *Br J Sports Med* 1998; **32**: 84.
25 Drotman DP. Professional boxing, bleeding and HIV testing. *JAMA* 1996; **276**: 193.
26 Federation Internationale de Medecine Sportive (FIMS). *Advice on HIV in Sport*. FIMS. 1996.
27 Thune I, Brenn T, Lund E, Gaard M. Physical activity and the risk of breast cancer. *N Engl J Med* 1997; **336**: 1269–73.
28 Woods JA, Davis JM. Exercise, monocyte/macrophage function and cancer. *Med Sci Sports Exer* 1994; **26**: 147–57.
29 Nash MS. Exercise and immunology. *Med Sci Sports Exer* 1994; **26**: 125–7.
30 Pedersen BK, Ullum H. NK response to physical activity: possible mechanisms of action. *Med Sci Sports Exer* 1994; **26**: 140–6.

21 Dermatological problems

Jock itch

This is not a new medical condition but is simply the athletes' term to describe tinea cruris. It is a fungal infection which thrives in a warm moist environment. It is found in skin folds of the groin sometimes extending along the upper thigh. It is itchy, and often has a raised margin typical of these infections. An athlete may be anxious that it is a more serious condition and reluctant to seek help. Treatment is simple, using topical antifungal agents, but the condition may recur due to re-infection or inadequate laundering of sports gear. With a troublesome infection the athlete should throw out their sporting underwear as it may be the source of the infection. Occasionally, an athlete may have used a steroid cream before seeking treatment. If this happens the infection can spread quite extensively and appear greatly out of control, but the treatment is the same and is effective.

Athlete's foot

Athlete's foot is also a fungal infection. It occurs between the toes, usually in the space between the 4th and 5th toes. Initially it causes an itchy pink rash with flaking of skin between the toes, but may become quite severe so that the skin is damp and macerated with large fissures. These fissures may become painful with bacterial superinfection. The feet should be kept clean and dry, and fungal infection alone can be treated with topical antifungal agents. Superinfection should be treated with antibacterials.

Other skin infections

Impetigo is a common bacterial skin infection. It is very contagious and easily spread among team-mates. Players should not share towels. The condition should be treated intensively with antibacterial agents and those with impetigo should not play contact sports.

A verruca is a wart-like lesion on the sole of the foot. The symptoms are due to pressure on the foot so that the verruca is pushed up into the skin of the sole of the foot. This may cause problems with pain and discomfort when the athlete attempts to run and gives the feeling of a stone in the shoe. It is common in the normal population, but because athletes share communal showers in changing rooms they are even more exposed to infection. Using 'flip-flops' or 'verruca socks' in the shower can offer some protection. Painless verrucas can be left alone and will eventually disappear. For troublesome verrucas the best approach is using topical treatments and a pummice stone. Using liquid nitrogen to cryofreeze the verruca can cause pain and discomfort and surgical removal is not now usually performed.

Herpes simplex

Herpes simplex is transmitted by close contact. It is the virus responsible for cold sores but this benign name disguises how it can produce a severe painful pustular facial infection with blisters and exudate. It is treated using modern topical antiviral agents, although often by the time the infection is manifest these agents are ineffective. For those who have recurrent infections, and who can sometimes feel a tingling before it occurs, treatment should be started as soon as possible. Oral versions of the antiviral agents are available but are not usually used in herpes simplex. Because of the nature of infection and its transmission, it may be spread by close contact such as in the rugby scrum or in wrestling, hence it attracts the name 'scrumpox' or 'herpes gladiatorum'. Those with a severe current herpes simplex infection should not play close contact sports.

Herpes simplex can be a problem in outdoor pursuits as it can be triggered by exposure to bright sunlight. Sun-blocks can be protective.

Eczema

Eczema is not a contraindication to exercise. Widespread flexural eczema may be a problem for the athlete who showers regularly using soap which can exacerbate the eczema, and the normal treatment regime of emolients and steroid creams can be difficult. Athletes can be confused by the word 'steroid' and should be reassured that there is no connection with anabolic steroids, which are prohibited drugs. There is no sanction on the use of topical steroid treatments. Foot eczema can occur as a reaction to footwear. This occurs most often on the dorsum, distal part of the foot, and responds to usual eczema treatment.

A common condition in the feet of athletes, although it occurs even more often among young people who wear runners and trainers as leisure shoes, is inflamed dry sore skin on the soles of the feet. If people wear runners constantly and the feet are sweaty, the skin becomes damp and macerated and later shiny and sore; this clears up if they wear alternative footwear which allows the feet to breathe.

Abrasion injuries

'Jogger's nipple' is an abrasion injury that occurs when the material in a running vest rubs roughly over the nipple. The injury can be prevented by wearing the appropriate clothing. Rough cotton or nylon should not be worn close to the skin and women should wear appropriate supportive underwear. Abrasion injuries can also be caused by the seams of running shorts and, in those with large thighs, from two legs rubbing together. Prevention is by wearing appropriate clothing. The treatment is to apply vaseline and allow the skin to heal. Hydrocortisone 1% cream may help speed recovery.

Psoriasis

Psoriasis is not a contraindication to sport, nor does sport influence the condition although the treatment can be messy and cause problems. Plantopustular psoriasis can cause confusion as patients may think it is associated with sportswear. Occasionally psoriatic arthritis causes joint pain and in the athlete the diagnosis can be confused by the high level of physical activity.

Sun screens

With increasing publicity about the damage that the sun can cause to the skin, athletes are becoming increasing aware of the need to use sun protection. This is especially important for those competing in parts of the world where the ozone layer is reduced, particularly in the Southern hemisphere. Athletes should wear appropriate clothing and use sunscreens. This includes the use of hats and long sleeved shirts but athletes should also protect the back of the neck and the legs. Many countries now announce skin burning times on their news bulletins and weather forecasts which is helpful but essentially sunburn causes skin damage and should be avoided.

Subungual haematoma

This can be very painful and cause considerable problems. It may occur due to trauma or when catching the toe awkwardly on the turf. Treatment can give almost instant relief and should be performed as soon as possible by releasing the blood clot. The nail is punctured either by drilling or by use of a hot trephine. (Some use a red hot expanded paperclip.) It may be accompanied by turf toe which is an acute sprain of the ligaments.

Blisters

Blisters are common. They occur when fluid gathers in the layers of the dermis as a reaction to friction. The fluid causes discomfort in the foot and is painful when running. Blisters also occur on the hands of those who grip, such as rowers. Blisters are usually deroofed with a sterile puncture. Eventually the skin hardens and becomes accustomed to the grip. Folk remedies to reduce blistering include the use of methylated spirits to harden the skin.

Sweat rash

One often hears the term 'sweat rash'. Originally used as a term to describe the prickly heat or miliaria that occurs in hot climates, it is a form of irritation of the sweat glands. There is no specific treatment but it is more likely to occur when clothing is made of a fabric that does not allow the skin the 'breathe' such as nylon and close fitting lycra type garments. There is no treatment other than to keep cool and change to cotton clothing. Clothing manufacturers have developed fabrics that help keep the skin dry and these may help. New yarns are incorporated in sports clothing, even socks.

Gravel rash

Gravel rash or road rash is a misnomer. It is a term used by cyclists to describe friction burns that occur when a cyclist falls and scrapes along the road surface taking off the top layer of skin. The skin may be torn off to varying levels, sometimes down to the muscle. 'Gravel rash' is common and since cyclists ride in such close formation in a bunch, if one falls, others inevitably fall too.

With mild friction burns there is merely loss of part of the superficial layer of skin which then forms an exudate. New skin grows from the lower layers underneath the exudate. With deeper friction burns the entire layer of skin is lost with no skin underneath to repair the damage. The damage heals from the edge of the wound and recovery is much slower. This new skin is not as supple and elastic as the original skin but is formed of scar tissue which is more rigid and more easily torn. Massaging moisturising cream into the scar tissue can improve suppleness.

When the skin is damaged, not only is the surface protective layer removed but the wound may be contaminated by pieces of gravel, glass, hay, cow dung and other detritus on the road. These contaminants must be removed to avoid infection and the wound should be cleaned with sterile water as soon as possible and dressed appropriately. To minimise injury, cyclists often wear two layers of clothing, so the two layers slide over each other when striking the road. Racing cyclists shave their legs and one possible benefit is that it prevents hairs sticking to the wound following a friction burn.

Suturing lacerations

If you are involved with an athlete or a team at the training or competition venue, you will almost certainly be asked to suture a laceration from time to time. These wounds may vary from a simple, small, clean laceration in the relatively clean environment of an indoor sport to a large, deep, jagged wound filled with mud and grass outdoors. There may be pressure from the athlete, other players and the manager to get the player back into the game as soon as possible. The doctor is expected to share this enthusiasm but touchline suturing may not always be in the player's best interest. Each decision should be made on its own merits and in the light of the knowledge and expertise of the doctor but one of the rules of medical practice is 'first do no harm' and this should guide any decision.

In suturing lacerations, every effort should be made to uphold standards in asepsis. A small clean uncontaminated laceration can easily be sutured with proper cleansing and aseptic technique. A large dirty wound requires far more attention and there is no place for inadequate care. This wound should be treated appropriately. If there is a well appointed first aid room, with good light, and equipment for proper wound toilet then it may be appropriate to suture the wound. But there are always the serious risks of tetanus, infection and scarring. The short-term gain of getting a player back on to the field of play may be off-set by the long-term risk.

The team doctor should, however, be prepared to cope with minor lacerations and carry a small suture pack to include a dressing pack, forceps, scissors, cleansing agents and sutures. It is often very inconvenient for an athlete, or away team, to go to an accident and emergency department for minor suturing and the athlete will always be very grateful if you can suture a laceration on the spot. Remember, however, to make appropriate medical notes, advise on tetanus immunisation if required, and arrange follow-up.

Ingrowing toenail

Hardly a sports injury, but certainly a condition that affects performance in sport. Although there are many theories, no-one really knows how or why ingrowing toenails occur. They do, however, cause problems because of pain and infection. When the edges of the nail grow deep into the tissue at the side of the nail they act as a foreign body and can become infected. This leaves the patient with a tender swollen infected messy toenail. Almost invariably ingrowing toenails occur on the big toe. They cause pain when walking, footwear may press on the toe, and kicking is almost impossible. The athlete is also afraid that someone may step on their toe, a major problem in contact sport. The initial treatment is with antibiotics, oral and topical, to reduce the infection but some operative procedure is usually necessary later. The operative management varies from simply trimming the nail to removal of the entire nail with sclerosis of the nailbed.

The simplest procedure to ease the pain of an ingrowing toenail can be undertaken by almost any general practitioner. Infection should be treated with antibiotics and when healed the edge of the nail can be removed. The toe should be anaesthetised by injecting approx 2–3 ml lignocaine 1%, on either side of the proximal toe to create a ring block. A tourniquet will reduce any blood loss. One blade of a small artery forcep can be pushed gently up under the side of the nail. This is closed and the nail is gently manoeuvred out of the deep gutter on the side of the nail. A small incision may be necessary on the skin at the base of the nail to allow the most proximal part to be released. The lateral part of the nail is then trimmed off and the incision sutured. The athlete can often play the next day without problems but using this procedure the ingrowing toenail can recur. Those who regularly undertake minor surgery will have their own favourite procedure for a more permanent improvement using one or a combination of wedge resection, nailbed removal or nailbed sclerosis.

22 Women and sport

Anatomical and physiological differences between men and women influence the relative difference in performance and the response to exercise. Women are smaller and tend to be of a different shape with a wider pelvis and narrower shoulders. They have less lean body mass and have a lower oxygen uptake capacity. In the sporting context these differences are significant in that they alter both the response to training and susceptibility to injury. Women have a greater proportion of body fat which means they have greater natural insulation and so retain heat more effectively. There are of course other important attributes of the woman athlete related to the menstrual cycle, menopause and postmenopausal osteoporosis.

Women are smaller by about 7%. They have proportionately shorter arms, so men have a mechanical advantage in sports such as throwing and tennis where terminal velocity is important. The female pelvis is wider which places the acetabula and hip joints more widely apart with greater angulation of the femur. This creates a greater 'Q' angle, which is the angle made by an imaginary line drawn from the anterior superior iliac spine to the midpoint of the patella crossing a vertical line drawn through the patella. With this greater 'Q' angle, the quadriceps muscle group tends to draw the patella laterally out of the patellofemoral groove so that women may be more susceptible to anterior knee pain, an overuse injury associated with some endurance sports.

Women have a greater proportion of body fat. The average sedentary male has 15% body fat compared to the average sedentary female with about 25%. These are population averages which may not apply to the sporting community where there is much greater variation depending on the sport and the different skills and body types. In those sports categorised by body weight, and in endurance sports where a low body weight increases the power-to-weight ratio, participants tend to have much lower body fat. In male endurance sports for example most participants have a body fat proportion of 8–10% with some recorded as low as 5%. In all sports, however, male competitors tend to have lower body fat than females, but this is not always an advantage and in events where heat conservation is important, long distance swimming for example, a greater body fat proportion is advantageous.

Menstrual cycle

Athletes in heavy training usually experience a reduction in the volume of menstrual loss and may even cease to have periods. Amenorrhoea is most common in runners, dancers and gymnasts and some believe that suppression of ovarian function in athletes is similar to that which occurs in postmenopausal women. It may be due low body fat, or to the effect of endurance training alone. Oestrogen is involved in bone metabolism and hypo-oestrogenic women may have impaired bone deposition. Osteoporosis is more a problem among thin women and is unusual in those who are overweight. It may be the high stress of training alone that affects the hypothalamic–pituitary axis. Peak bone mass occurs in the third decade, so if there is reduction in calcium deposition at this age, this may lead to later problems with osteoporosis. There is some oestrogen metabolism (aromatisation) in fat or adipose tissue.

General practitioners should be aware of other possible causes of amenorrhoea and not simply attribute amenorrhoea to sport. Pregnancy is, of course, the most common cause, but more unusual causes include polycystic ovarian disease, hyperprolactinaemia and some neoplasms.

Amenorrhoea should be investigated and, in the absence of any other causes, it should be treated with combined oestrogen and progesterone, calcium and vitamin D, and advice to the athlete to increase their weight. There is also evidence that heavy training in youth can delay the menarche in some cases by up to 2 years.

Among women athletes exceptionally low body fat can lead to problems. Low body weight is often associated with menstrual cycle disturbance, so that in endurance sports, where low body weight is of particular advantage through altering the power–weight ratio, and where competitors have body fat as low as

12% or less, the menstrual cycle may cease altogether. While this may be of some potential benefit to the athlete, whose training is not now inconvenienced by menstruation, there is increasing recognition of the long-term risks associated with changes in bone metabolism. Bone deposition, which is regulated by oestrogen, may be reduced in thin amenorrhoiec athletes with an increased incidence of stress fractures in the short-term, and the long-term development of osteoporosis. These effects are not confined to sport alone, and one group of performers who have very similar problems are dancers. In one study [1] of professional female dancers those with a history of delayed menarche and amenorrhoea were found to have a decrease in lumbar spine bone mineral density. Interestingly, there appeared to be a partial protective effect from weight-bearing on bone mineral density of the femoral neck. These features of low body weight, amenorrhoea and osteoporosis are now known as the female athletic triad.

The cause of this menstrual disturbance has been debated and may or may not be related to sport. In some athletes, gymnasts and lightweight rowers, amenorrhoea may be associated with very low body weight and its effect on oestrogen metabolism. Alternatively the stress of high intensity training and racing may directly influence the hypothalamus, perhaps mediated through cortisol. Interestingly, high intensity sport has also been shown to have an effect on male testosterone levels [2].

Paradoxically, while low body weight and the related hormonal changes associated with high intensity athletic training in younger years can lead to osteoporosis, there is considerable evidence of benefit from weight-bearing activity in protecting against osteoporosis in the older woman. Walking, for example, can increase spinal bone density in postmenopausal women [3], but these benefits are not restricted to aerobic activities and there is also evidence that resistance exercise can have similar advantages, even in a programme of only 45 minutes per session on 2 days per week [4]. Indeed, high impact exercise over 18 months can also improve bone mass, muscle strength and other fitness parameters in healthy premenopausal women [5]. Improvements in bone mineral density of 1–3% have been shown in resistance and aerobic-type exercise, but this study of high impact exercise demonstrated gains of 1.4–3.7%. It may be that the loading effect of skeletal impact causes greater increase in bone mineral density. This would be in keeping with observations in amenorrhoiec women gymnasts who have higher bone mineral density [6] compared to similarly amenorrhoiec runners.

The benefits associated with exercise are of advantage to all women, because osteoporosis is a widespread problem affecting about 25% of women over the age of 50 years, and up to 50% of those over the age of 75 years with the risk of fractures of the spine, wrist and femur greatest in postmenopausal years. It is likely that the incidence and cost of osteoporotic fractures will increase [7] with an ageing population. Many factors are associated with falls leading to fractures and among these aetiological factors are balance, reflexes, muscle strength and power of the legs [8]. It is possible even to improve strength, functional status and mobility in nursing home residents with multiple pathology [9,10].

Bone mineral density is the major protective factor and many studies confirm the importance of physical activity in improving bone mass and hence bone strength. It is important, however, that this activity be weight bearing. Physical fitness can also aid strength, reaction time, balance and coordination, and these also help to reduce falls. All these beneficial effects are likely to disappear if training is not continued so that exercise must become part of the lifestyle.

Bone mineral density loss is a feature of women athletes but there are also changes in bone mineral content and lean body mass in male athletes [11]. This decreased bone mineral density in men is as a result of calcium loss in sweat and skin but can be prevented by calcium intake during intense exercise.

There are additional benefits from physical activity in women. Obesity is a well-known risk factor for breast cancer but recent evidence from Norway has shown that physical activity has some protective effect. In a study of 25,624 women aged 20–54 followed over a 14-year period, of whom 350 developed invasive breast cancer, it was shown that women who took regular exercise had a risk of breast cancer that was only two thirds of that in women whose work and leisure was spent in sedentary occupation [12]. The benefit of exercise in increasing longevity is also seen in postmenopausal women. In a huge study of 40,417 women aged 55–69 years over 7 years, the risk of death decreased in a dose–response relationship with the exercise taken. Those who exercised most, in terms of frequency and intensity, had a 30% lower risk of death from all causes compared to those who exercised least. Moderate exercise had a 22% lower risk of death [13].

Athletic performance

Women do not perform as well as men in most athletic events. There may be a number of reasons for this, related to both the anatomical differences between men and women and the nature of most competitive events. Historically most sporting events had their origin in the traditional hunting and warrior role, where men had a natural advantage, so that as sporting events evolved, they tended to favour male attributes. Physiological parameters of athletic men and women reflect these differences so that women tend to have lower values for VO_2max which, even when corrected for lean body mass, remains at about 70–75% of men. This may in part be due to their lower haemoglobin level (men $15.8 \, gl^{-1}$ and women $13.9 \, gl^{-1}$) but also due to their relatively smaller hearts. In sprint events, power which is related to muscle mass is the key to performance and this in turn is determined by testosterone.

In contrast, women have advantages in some sports. They have a lower centre of gravity so that they tend to have better balance and hence excel on the beam apparatus in gymnastics (not a men's event). Their greater body fat proportion tends to give them an advantage in heat conservation so that they have an advantage in events such as ultra long-distance swimming.

The differences in performance may also be because women have not traditionally taken part in sport, and women's sport is at an earlier evolutionary stage. Women have only been competing in athletics since the First World War and when women applied to compete in the Olympics their requests were turned down repeatedly. Eventually women organised their own events in 1922, 1926, 1930 and 1934. Women were allowed to compete in five events in the 1928 Olympics, one of which was the 800 m. Some competitors collapsed during the event and as a result the 800 m did not reappear until 32 years later. It was believed that women were unable to cope with the physiological stress of such events. Women's distance events are a relatively recent phenomenon and the 3000 m event was only introduced into the European Championships in 1974, the marathon into world championships in 1983, and only in 1984 did the Olympics include a marathon event for women. What is interesting, however, is the rate at which women's performance in sport has improved and that the rate of increase is much greater than that of men. Extrapolating these results forward suggests that women will soon overtake men in sporting prowess.

The effect of the menstrual cycle on performance

The menstrual cycle, with the build up of oestrogen towards ovulation and subsequent decline with elevation of progesterone, can have a major physical and psychological impact on some women. Some athletes feel that these cyclical changes affect their athletic performance. Menstruation, and the premenstrual syndrome, can cause problems with the physical symptoms of weight gain, painful breasts, abdominal distension and, of course, dysmenorrhoea. Others may have tiredness, irritability, and sometimes insomnia and increased feelings of anxiety.

The effect of the menstrual cycle on many parameters including accidents, examination results and crime is well documented but research on athletes and their performance shows variable results. When asked to give an assessment of their performance in training over a number of cycles, for example, athletes reported perceived performance as best at the time of and shortly after ovulation and perceived performance declined towards menstruation. Sensing that the menstrual cycle could alter performance, athletes began to manipulate the cycle so that menstruation did not coincide with major competition. While this had some advantages, some athletes felt that, while avoiding dips in performance, they did not experience the corresponding highs.

Exercise and pregnancy

Some believe that pregnancy can improve subsequent sporting performance. There are many examples of athletes who have performed better following return to competition after pregnancy but little objective evidence. If so, and it will be difficult to prove, there are a number of possible reasons why this could be so. Some believe that the cardiovascular stress of carrying the baby has a training effect. Others suggest a different pathway and that in the gifted athlete who has competed all her life, the enforced rest associated with pregnancy allows the athlete to return refreshed and enthusiastic for the sport. The mechanism may be psychological. Nevertheless some athletes plan pregnancy to fit in with training programmes.

Athletes may also ask if they should exercise during pregnancy. There are few contraindications to training during in pregnancy, although there are practical difficulties in the third trimester.

Many athletes try to remain active and being fit allows the pregnant mother to cope better with the progressive incapacity of pregnancy. A major prospective longitudinal cohort study of 398 pregnant women found that those who were more physically active had fewer adverse symptoms associated with pregnancy [14,15]. In this study there were no differences in morbidity, extended hospital stay or lower birth weight when comparing physically active and inactive mothers. Those who have been active tend to have a lower risk of toxaemia, varicose veins, piles, depression and insomnia. They have fewer stretch marks and shorter less tiring labour, with fewer complications, and more rapid recovery from labour. Pregnancy may influence the choice and intensity of sport especially with increasing abdominal size which limits mobility. Ligaments become looser and pubic symphysis problems can prevent any activity. It unrealistic, however, to try to maintain the same level of training as before pregnancy. Some activities are contraindicated such as horse riding, diving and waterskiing. If exercise is anaerobic there is a theoretical risk of foetal hypoxia and in endurance sport there may be a risk to the foetus from the inevitable rise in core body temperature. The suggestion that there may be a reduction in uterine blood flow with exercise is less convincing.

Gender testing

If men have an inherent advantage in most of the established sports, then it is important to ensure that sport is fair and that women can compete with equals. This means creating separate categories for men and women and ensuring that men do not cheat! This is not as easy as it may appear at first and appearance is not always the most accurate test of gender. There are celebrated examples of famous female athletes who were subsequently discovered to be male. Stella Walasiewicz won the women's 100 yds gold at the 1932 Olympics but was found to be male after her death in a gang shoot-out in the USA, and Dora (later Herman) Ratjen won the high jump in 1936. In recognition of this problem, gender assessment using visual inspection of athletes was introduced at the 1966 European Athletic Championships. At this event 243 women athletes were inspected by a panel of doctors. Later that year, at the Commonwealth Games in Jamaica, this examination included digital examination. Gender verification was an unpleasant and difficult experience for the athlete and there were efforts to identify alternative methods. The sex chromatin test was first used at the 1967 Winter Olympics and at the 1968 Summer Olympics. The test is carried out by examining cells taken from a buccal mucosa smear. The genetic female XX chromosone configuration leaves a redundant X chromosone appearing as a black dot known as the 'Barr body' in female cells. This test was not intended to be definitive and was to be used only in screening so that if there were insufficient Barr bodies visible, the athlete should be offered formal karyotype and gynaecological assessment. To fail a 'sex test' has a devastating effect on an athlete. While further assessment may identify those who were unfairly excluded, the trauma of the initial test result is such that few have gone forward for karyotype and examination. Data published in 1991 indicated that 13 women had been excluded from competition on the basis of sex chromatin testing between 1972 and 1990 [16].

International competitors have a registration card which they must show at major events but they only require a certificate for competition when they attain a high level of performance in sport and are candidates for international selection. If an athlete cannot be issued with a certificate they cannot perform in female competition, but the psychological trauma of coming to terms with this gender uncertainty can be much more disturbing than the sporting implications.

There was dissatisfaction with the sex chromatin test. It is subject to human error and there are huge implications associated with false positive and false negative tests. A new gender verification was introduced at the Albertville and Barcelona Olympic Games in 1992 [17]. This test uses polymerase chain reaction (PCR) to amplify DNA from buccal cells so that the SRY gene, a testis determining gene, could be detected on the Y chromosone if present. This test is a vast improvement but even if it is 99% accurate, it may still give an inaccurate result in a proportion of competitors at any major event.

Chromosone testing is not absolute and gender is determined by many factors [18]. The main question is if participation should be determined by phenotype or genotype. People with chromosome abnormalities such as Turner's syndrome XO are female but would fail the test, although it is unlikely that someone with Turner's syndrome would become an athlete of standing. People with Kleinfelter's XXY would pass the test although male. Leaving aside chromosome anomalies, testicular feminising syndrome is a condition where there is target organ insensitivity to normal androgens so that those affected may have testes but have the outward appearance of being female. Other conditions such as congenital adrenal hyperplasia, androblastoma, and to a much lesser extent polycystic ovarian syndrome, raise endogenous androgens which may lead to a more masculine appearance. The difficulties associated with gender verification are complex and are as much associated with our perceptions of femininity as scientific testing. Realising the difficulties associated with gender verification, there is consensus in favour of abandoning gender verification [19,20].

References

1 Keay N, Fogelman I, Blake G. Bone mineral density in professional female dancers. *Br J Sports Med* 1997; **31**: 143–7.
2 Bennell KL, Brickner PD, Malcolm SA. Effect of altered reproductive function and lowered testosterone levels on bone density in male endurance athletes. *Br J Sports Med* 1996; **30**: 205–8.
3 Nelson M, Fisher E, Dilmanian F *et al*. A one year walking programme and increased dietary calcium in post menopausal women – effects on bone. *Am J Clin Nutr* 1991; **53**: 1304–11.
4 Nelson ME, Fiatarone MA, Morganti CM *et al*. Effects of high intensity strength training on multiple risk factors for osteoporotic fractures. *JAMA* 1994; **272**: 1909–14.
5 Heinonen A, Kannus P, Sioevanen H *et al*. Randomised controlled trial of effect of high impact exercise on selected risk factors for osteoporotic fractures. *Lancet* 1996; **348**: 1343–47.
6 Robinson TL, Snow-Harter C, Taffe DR *et al*. Gymnasts exhibit higher bone mass than runners despite similar prevalence of amenorrhoea. *J Bone Min Res* 1995; **10**: 26–35.
7 Kannus P, Parkkari J, Niemi S. Age adjusted incidence of hip fractures. *Lancet* 1995; **346**: 50–51.
8 Drinkwater BL, Grimston SK, Raab-Cullen DM, Snowharter CM. ACSM position stand on osteoporosis and exercise. *Med Sci Sports Exer* 1995; **27**: i–vii.
9 Tinettii ME, Liu WL, Claus EV. Predictors and prognosis of inability to get up after falls in elderly persons. *JAMA* 1993; **269**: 65–67.
10 Tinetti ME, Baker DI, McAvay G *et al*. A multifactorial intervention to reduce the risk of falling among elderly people living in the community. *N Engl J Med* 1994; **331**: 821–7.
11 Kleseges RC, Ward KD, Shelton ML *et al*. Changes in bone mineral content and lean body mass in male athletes; mechanisms of action and intervention effects. *JAMA* 1996; **276**: 226–30.
12 Thune I, Brenn T, Lund E, Gaard M. Physical activity and the risk of breast cancer. *N Engl J Med* 1997; **336**: 1269–73.
13 Kushi LH, Fee RM, Folsom AR *et al*. Physical activity and mortality in postmenopausal women. *JAMA* 1997; **277**: 1287–92.
14 Sternfield B, Quesenberry CP Jr, Eskenazi B, Newman LA. Exercise and pregnancy outcomes. *Med Sci Sports Exer* 1995; **27**: 634–40.

15 Clapp JF III, Capeless EL. Neonatal morphometrics after endurance exercise during pregnancy. *Am J Obstet Gynecol* 1990; **163**: 1605–11

16 Ferguson-Smith MA, Ferris EA. Gender verification in sport: the need for change? *Br J Sports Med* 1991; **25**: 17–21.

17 Serrat A, deHerreros AG. Gender verification in sports by PCR amplification of SRY and DYZ1 Y chromosome specific sequences: presence of DYZ1 repeat in female athletes. *Br J Sports Med* 1996; **30**: 305–9.

18 Puffer JC. Gender verification; a concept whose time has come and passed? *Br J Sports Med* 1996; **30**: 278.

19 Ljungqvist A, Simpson J. Medical examination for health of all athletes replacing the need for gender verification in international sports: the International Amateur Athletic Federation Plan. *JAMA* 1992; **267**: 850–52.

20 Simpson J, Ljungqvist A, de la Chapelle A *et al*. Gender verification and the next Olympic Games. *JAMA* 1993; **269**: 357–8.

23 Diet and sport

Athletes are particularly aware of the importance of diet and will often ask about food, fluid and dietary supplements. They are conscious of the importance of what they eat and how it can affect performance, but also readily accept suggestions for faddy diets and dietary supplements for performance enhancement. While they often have a very good understanding of exercise physiology they may have little understanding of energy metabolism.

Diet is important for sport, and indeed may make the difference in performance. Finding the correct dietary balance is important but the greatest difference between athletes and the sedentary population is the quantity of food required. The athletes' greatly increased calorie needs are due to their increased energy expenditure, but, because of the time spent preparing, training and competing, there is less time to buy, prepare and consume the correct food. Most athletes have some idea of what constitutes the correct diet, but it is much more difficult to ensure that the correct diet is available so that dietary problems can easily occur. While they may also have some theoretical knowledge, they may need some advice on how they may translate this into practice. The main focus should be on diet during training, and in particular during the periods of heaviest training in endurance athletes. Energy supply during training and the ability to recover after training are the key to gaining the most from training. Diet during competition is perhaps less critical.

Carbohydrates when metabolised produce 4 kcal per gram. Carbohydrates can be classified into two groups: the sugars (simple carbohydrates) such as glucose, sucrose and lactose, and starches (complex carbohydrates) such as flour, potatoes and cereal. An active sportsperson should eat a diet containing 60–70% of their total calorie intake as carbohydrate which is about 500–650 g of carbohydrate per day. These are metabolised to produce glycogen, the energy substrate used in cellular metabolism, hence the importance of the high carbohydrate diet to the athlete who requires an efficient energy source for sustained muscle activity. The so-called simple carbohydrates are in highly processed foods in which the constituent sugars are easily available and provide a very rapid source of energy. They are sometimes described as empty calories because of the lack of vitamins, minerals and fibre. Complex carbohydrates provide energy as nature stores it, together with vitamins and minerals in vegetables, fruits and cereal crops. The athlete may have a problem in meeting the additional energy requirements. It is often impossible or impractical to consume their high calorie requirement only in the form of complex carbohydrate and there is a place in an athlete's diet for some additional simple calories from confectionery, cakes and soft drinks.

Protein rich foods include fish, meat and eggs, and 4 kcal is available from each gram of protein. By eating a normal balanced diet most athletes consume sufficient protein, which should constitute 10–15% of total energy intake. While muscle is predominantly protein, a high protein diet is not necessary for muscle development. Protein is metabolised to its constituent amino acids. There are 21 amino acids of which 8 are known as the essential amino acids. A balanced diet should contain adequate protein and supply all the amino acids. Complete foods such as meat and fish include all the essential amino acids, but vegetarians may require supplements. One of the difficulties with protein-rich foods is that they often contain a lot of fat. It is best to trim excess fat off meat dishes.

Athletes often ask if they need extra protein because they are training. There is an increased protein requirement of about 7 gram per day above the normal basic requirement of 25 gram for an athlete in training. In the average diet, about 10% of the calories are supplied as protein, so that the normal dietary intake usually exceeds even this additional requirement in training. Vast quantities of protein are therefore not required in the diet and protein supplements are unnecessary.

Dietary fat is a concentrated energy source, providing 9 kcal per gram, but unfortunately it is a very inefficient energy source. The proportion of fat in the diet should be 25–30% of total dietary intake but fats are often hidden in the diet and people may not be aware of the fat content of common foods. Most people are aware of the fat in butter, cheese, spreads and cooking oil but less aware of the high fat content in crisps, chocolate, biscuits and cakes. In aerobic metabolism one litre of oxygen releases 5 kcal from carbohydrate but only 4.7 kcal from fat. This small difference is very important to performance. Although excess dietary fat is discouraged, some dietary fat is essential for many body activities.

A typical high carbohydrate diet should include: bread, potatoes, pasta, rice, noodles, breakfast cereal, porridge. Fruit and vegetables also provide a high carbohydrate energy source packaged with fibre and vitamins as nature intended. Sugars are also a high energy carbohydrate energy source and have a place as a high calorie supplements in those who use a lot of energy. It would be difficult to consume 6,000 or more calories in a high fibre diet alone so high energy sugars, in food or drinks, have a place. Convenience foods usually have a high fat content, which is unfortunate because these may form a major part of the diet of some athletes who, when training intensely, do not have the time to buy and prepare the correct food. Take away food: chips, pizza, burgers etc. have a high fat content as do confectionery and cakes. Drinks are a useful energy source and are especially important in fluid replacement. During long intensity training or racing, drinks are an ideal energy source.

Muscle energy metabolism

Glycogen is the key energy source used in exercise. Most glycogen is stored in the liver although some is present in the muscle cell. The quantity of stored glycogen is sufficient for about 2 hours of sustained muscle activity. We can illustrate the limitations of this energy source through the example of what happens during a marathon run. A moderately good runner, exercising vigorously, will have reached about 20 miles by 2 hours, and have consumed their entire glycogen supply. At about this time they sense they have run out of energy, muscles tire, they feel fatigued and feel unable to go another step. This is the 'wall', a purely physiological event. The elite marathon runner, however, seldom feels this way and has difficulty understanding what people mean by this 'wall'. One important feature of endurance training is its effect in subtly shifting metabolism to include some fat utilisation. The elite marathon runner can therefore eke their energy supply out longer than the 2 hours expected because of the combination of carbohydrate and fat metabolism and they never 'hit the wall'.

In an effort to avoid this glycogen depletion, athletes began to experiment with glycogen loading. In the early versions of the glycogen loading diet there was a glycogen depletion stage. During this phase the athlete progressively depleted the muscle cells by exercising but consuming a low carbohydrate diet. The athlete felt very fatigued but their cells were 'hungry for glycogen'. The second phase was the glycogen loading phase where they consumed excess carbohydrate in order that the cells would super compensate. In theory this should supply extra energy substrate for the event. Glycogen is best replaced by consuming carbohydrate, hence the tradition of the pasta party prior to the marathon. The glycogen depletion phase is now considered unnecessary, and athletes simply reduce the intensity of training and increase the carbohydrate proportion of their diet in anticipation of a major event. One unexpected side-effect of this diet was the increase in body weight prior to the event. With glycogen depletion the body weight falls and with supercompensation body weight climbs again as each gram of glycogen stores three grams of water so some athletes feel very sluggish before the event.

Related to the glycogen depletion phase of the diet is unintentional glycogen depletion that can occur in endurance athletes who train excessively without an adequate diet or rest. Training hard every day reduces glycogen stores, but without rest these stores do not recover. By the end of 5–7 days the glycogen stores are depleted and the athlete is exhausted. It requires 48 hours for the muscle glycogen stores to recover after a long duration intense training session. Dieticians recommend a high fibre complex carbohydrate diet. Common sense dictates that such a diet would be too bulky and athletes often supplement their diet with high energy foods.

The metabolic load of a high intensity event sustained over a number of days, such as occurs in the Tour de France or trans Atlantic rowing, is exceptional and there are immense difficulties in matching the energy needs. One of the features that separates the successful athlete in such an event is the ability to match the energy load with energy intake. If one is losing weight then clearly one is not in energy balance, so the successful athlete should complete such an event without significant weight loss.

Glycogen stores are best restored in the period immediately after training or competition. In endurance events, especially cycle stage races where there are repeated daily competitions, the competitor should aim to eat some carbohydrate, in the form of a high calorie fluid or light carbohydrate meal, as soon as possible after each stage.

Vitamins are essential nutrients required in very small quantities and which are necessary for specific functions. They cannot be manufactured and must be supplied in the diet. There are 13 known vitamins of which vitamins A,D,K, and E are fat soluble. They are stored in the liver, with sufficient stores for a few months. The remainder are water soluble and include vitamin C and the B vitamins: thiamine B1, riboflavin, niacin, biotin, pantothenic acid, pyridoxine B6, folate, cyanocobalmin B12. In most cases normal food contains sufficient vitamins and there is no need for supplementation. If an athlete consumes their additional calories in a balanced diet then there is no need for vitamin supplementation. While excess water-soluble vitamins are excreted in the urine, there is a potential risk from excess fat-soluble vitamin ingestion.

Minerals such as iron, potassium, calcium, sodium, zinc, magnesium and others are required in small quantity. There is considerable medical interest in their importance at present. Sodium is important in fluid balance and some of the other minerals and trace elements have a role in aerobic metabolism. Iron is essential for production of haemoglobin and myoglobin. Measurement of haemoglobin is not straightforward in athletes and the measured haemoglobin content can vary quite markedly depending on the phase of training and timing of the blood sample. Haemoconcentration can occur in those who are dehydrated, while haemodilution may occur quite naturally in endurance athletes. Iron deficiency anaemia can occur, however, and is an easily remediable cause of impaired performance. Iron studies, to include iron and ferritin levels, should be a routine part of the athlete's assessment and low iron levels do tend to impair performance, even in the absence of anaemia. Iron supplements may often be required and athletes should be advised how excess tea and coffee impair absorption of iron, but how vitamin C and fruit juices can improve absorption. Iron deficiency anaemia, especially among athletes, is also becoming more common because of the decreased consumption of red meat.

Making the weight

In many sports competitors are graded into weight categories. In boxing, judo and weight lifting there are a number of weight categories. In rowing there are two grades, lightweight and open, but in horseracing it is an advantage to be as light as possible. In sports where body weight is carried, distance running in particular, the advantage is with those who are lightest but who have the greatest endurance fitness. One can improve fitness by training, but athletes also realise that they can improve performance by altering the other side of the equation through loss of body weight. Efforts to lose body weight, together with very high training loads can border on the obsessive, even pathological. Dancers too have similar body weight problems, but their focus is on aesthetic factors and the need to have a certain body shape to be successful.

Clearly common sense determines that athletes should be able to predict their competition weight and prepare for this appropriately. One means of predicting possible weight loss is through estimates of body composition using skinfold thickness tests. But there are problems, athletes may not adhere to planned weight reduction programmes through the off season, or they may be still growing. They may then resort to dehydration and starvation in order to make the weight. The temptation is always to try to squeeze an athlete down to compete in the lowest weight category possible. This is done in the short term by dehydration and weight loss of up to 3 kg by dehydration is not unknown.

The pre-event meal

Competitors in many sports worry about what constitutes the most appropriate pre-event meal. Not a lot of benefit is gained by the food consumed in the final hours before competition but all can be lost by a mistake. The endurance athlete should approach the event having made an appropriate training taper and diet adjustment so their glycogen stores are complete. No additional food intake is likely to greatly improve performance so there is no need for a last-minute urgency to eat more. One's pre-event meal should be sufficient only to keep away the pangs of hunger.

The content and timing of the meal are important. Foods that are poorly or slowly digested should be avoided. Protein is digested slowly and both fat and protein are inappropriate for use as an energy source for sport. Gastric emptying will be slowed too by precompetition stress and anxiety. The most appropriate pre-event meal is a light carbohydrate meal of perhaps bread, pasta, potatoes and vegetables. Protein and fat (including chocolate) should be avoided. The meal should be consumed at least 3 hours before the event.

 If an athlete is competing through the day with perhaps heats and finals, they may need some carbohydrate intake through the day and will require additional fluid. Both purposes are best served by a simple carbohydrate drink. One should remember that warm drinks are poorly absorbed. The drink most suitable depends on the balance between fluid and calorie requirement. Most sports drinks have very similar contents and there may be little to choose between them. The most important factor is that the athlete is prepared to drink them so palatability is the key. More concentrated high calorie carbohydrate drinks are slowly absorbed but more suitable in cool conditions, while a less concentrated more easily absorbed fluid is more suitable in warm conditions. When competing in endurance sports, many athletes find that their taste and drink preference is altered. Drinks with relatively high glucose content, which tasted fine while resting, are sickly and unpleasant when competing. What may taste fine in normal circumstances may be impossible to drink while exercising. It is essential that athletes, especially those competing in endurance sports, try out various drinks available while mimicking race conditions.

Post-event diet

Glycogen stores are best replaced immediately after an endurance event. There may also be a fluid deficit. Replacing fluid and glycogen are a priority if the athlete is to compete or train intensely the following day. The athlete should aim to consume a high carbohydrate snack as soon as possible after the event together with substantial fluid intake. This should be planned beforehand as it may be some time after the event before the athlete has a formal meal, either at home or, if competing away, at the team hotel. Suitable snacks, aiming for a minimum of 50 g carbohydrate would include bread and bananas/honey/jam. The post-event meal should also be a high carbohydrate meal with adequate fluid replacement. Team management should ensure that adequate drinks are always available.

Dietary supplements

Athletes are susceptible to suggestion of benefit from dietary supplements. Many will be taking extra vitamins and iron.

There are many marketed supplements including standard carbo-hydrate and protein supplements, amino acid powders and other products such as chromium picolinate, L-carnithine, inosine and co-enzyme Q. There is some basis to the use of antioxidant sup-plements, not as an ergogenic aid, but more for general health. Others will be attracted by the claims made on behalf of dietary supplements such as Ginseng although there is little objective evidence of benefit. Creatine is a newer ergogenic aid, which has some support from research evidence.

Antioxidants

Vitamin C has a protective effect against atherogenesis [1] and it is possible that some of the health benefits of exercise could be mediated through increased antioxidants. Vitamin C is a power-ful antioxidant which acts as a scavenger for free radicals. Physical exercise, in spite of its beneficial effect may also increase the leakage of free radicals, especially at high levels. Intense exer-cise may lead to oxidative stress with possible lipid peroxidation of polyunsaturated fatty acids in cell membranes. If the level of exercise is such that the level of free radicals exceeds the scaven-ger effect it is arguable that those at the highest levels of physical activity should have antioxidant supplementation. In a recent population survey, there was no relationship between physical activity and ascorbate level [2]. Similarly there was no association with another method of estimating antioxidant potential, the cal-culated TRAP [3] or with vitamin E [4]. As would be expected, smokers had lower ascorbate levels. In the general population there is no evidence of a need for vitamin C supplementation, although there may be a case for supplements in those who are most active.

Ginseng is a title used to describe a number of preparations which include Chinese or Korean ginseng, American ginseng, Japanese ginseng and Russian ginseng, all different but all vari-eties of the plant *Araliaceae*. These products are sold as health supplements to give extra energy or as tonics with a remarkable list of reported benefits. There is little research evidence of a benefit to athletic performance. There is a potential hazard, how-ever, in that some ginseng preparations may contain significant quantities of ephedrine, a stimulant included on the list of drugs prohibited by the IOC.

Creatine

The intracellular energy source for short-acting muscle contraction is phosphocreatine (PCr). This led to the belief that creatine supplementation may help prevent depletion and hence reduce fatigue in short-duration high-intensity muscle activity. There is some basis for this belief but the evidence is not yet clear [5]. There is evidence that creatine can help maintain performance [6] in short-duration maximal exercise but it seems that there are some athletes who do not gain benefit from supplementation.

Caffeine is well known to improve performance, but quantities sufficient to have a significant effect on performance are likely to produce urine concentrations in excess of the permitted urine sample threshold under the rules of doping of the IOC.

Fluid balance

Maintaining fluid balance should be a major priority for the athlete. In sport we generate heat and the major means of losing heat is by evaporation through sweating. Sweat loss in endurance sports in moderate climates is within the range 1–1.5 litre/hour so strategies for fluid replacement are important. In most cases fluid loss in moderate climates can be replaced easily by consuming extra fluid, but unless the athlete is aware of the need for fluid replacement they may become progressively dehydrated.

Dehydration can be a problem for those who compete in weight category sports and who deliberately use dehydration as a strategy to make the weight. When dehydrated their heat loss mechanism may be impaired which is especially important in endurance sports. In lightweight rowing for example there is inadequate time between the weigh-in and the race to replace fluid loss. In addition, the rower may be reluctant to rehydrate if they know they have to weigh-in the following morning. Performance in rowing, a high intensity endurance sport, will always be impaired when dehydrated. Even a moderate level of dehydration, of 2%, can impair performance. The problem is not quite so important in explosive sports where heat loss may not be so critical. Training and competing in hot and humid conditions are a particular problem and there must be a carefully planned strategy and acclimatisation programme when travelling to countries where the temperature and humidity are high.

References

1 Horsey J, Livesley B, Dickenson JWT. Ischemic heart disease and aged patients: effects of ascorbic acid on lipoproteins. *J Hum Nutr* 1981; **35**: 53–8.
2 Sharpe PC, MacAuley D, Mc Crum EE *et al*. Vitamin C and exercise in the Northern Ireland Population. *Int J Vit Nutr Res* 1994; **64**: 277–82.
3 Sharpe PC, Duly EB, MacAuley D *et al*. Total radical trapping antioxidant potential (TRAP) and exercise. *Q J Med* 1996; **89**: 223–8.
4 Duly EB, Trinnick TR, Kennedy DG *et al*. Vitamin E and the Northern Ireland Population. *Ann Clin Biochem* 1996; **33**: 234–40.
5 Greenhalf PL. Creatine supplementation: recent developments. *Br J Sports Med* 1996; **30**: 276–7.
6 Greenhalf PL, Casey A, Short AH *et al*. Influence of oral creatine supplementation on muscle torque during repeated bouts of maximal voluntary exercise in man. *Clin Sci* 1993; **843**: 565–71.

24 Drugs in sport

Hardly a week goes by without some new allegation, revelation or appeal against the accusation of the use of drugs in sport. Athletes have always sought that extra advantage, and competitors have been tempted to use drugs to assist performance even as far back as the early Greek Olympics. Certain drugs can help performance and the problem is unlikely to go away [1]. It is likely that athletes will continue to use drugs to enhance performance and there is a continuing struggle between the sporting organisations in their attempt to control the abuse of drugs, and the athletes and their colleagues who continually seek new drugs and methods to confound the tests. In the past, sport may have been a matter of personal and national prestige but now the rewards of success are huge and competitors in many sports are professional. Even at local and regional level, athletes train and compete full-time and sport is their only source of income. Without making any moral judgement, or comment from a medical perspective, one can easily understand the pressure to seek any advantage. Competitors undertake very intense and sustained training and are encouraged to take a scientific approach to all aspects of preparation. In seeking every scientific advantage in nutrition, fluid replacement, physiological preparation and medical support, it is not difficult to understand how the lines between what is permitted and what is prohibited can become blurred. Sporting organisations try to enforce the rules, but the rules themselves seem open to interpretation and the penalties for breaking the rules are hardly a major deterrent. The picture changes too with the drugs of abuse and the drug users seem to be always just one step ahead.

Some athletes believe that drugs are of benefit in training and competition. There is circumstantial evidence from performance records and empirical evidence that they are an aid to performance but there is little objective research evidence to support this view. It would be foolish, however, to use this lack of evidence as proof of lack of effect. The belief that drugs are effective is so strong among some groups of athletes that they believe they could not compete without pharmacological assistance. It is interesting to contrast these views, beliefs and understandings with the current move towards evidence-based medicine and, in theory, we ought to be able to advise patients and athletes based on the latest research findings. There is very little research available. The use of performance enhancing drugs in sport is prohibited and undertaking proper methodologically sound research is almost impossible. The findings in any literature search are therefore unlikely to give us any reasonable indication either of the prevalence or effectiveness of performance enhancing drugs. The first evidence to confirm the effectiveness of therapeutic doses of anabolic steroids was published recently, but it is unlikely that we will build up an extensive research portfolio.

From a general practice perspective there are likely to be two main problems. We may be dealing with athletes, within the normal practice population, who compete at the highest level and are subject to dope testing. Some of the medications used in normal medical practice, while they have a minimal performance enhancing effect, are prohibited under the doping regulations. Athletes may also enquire about other medications and aids to performance available 'over the counter' to ensure that they do not contain prohibited medications. In these circumstances, we do not wish to lead the athlete unwittingly into an inadvertent positive drug test. The second potential problem is in caring for those athletes who are taking performance enhancing drugs and understanding their effect on the general health and well-being of the patient. These medications have both physical and psychological side-effects which can affect not just the athlete, but also their family. Sporting organisations have a further problem in attempting to detect those who take performance enhancing drugs and who may deliberately set out to beat the testing system.

Banned drugs

General practitioners should have access to the list of prohibited substances. An up-to-date list is printed in the British National Formulary (BNF) and doctors and patients have immediate access to this list. It may be difficult, however, to determine from a chemical name if a drug is prohibited. While the list is comprehensive it includes the term 'and related substances' which may not help with some drug names. Those in doubt should contact the Sports Council who have a very useful list of those medications permitted for use in athletes. They publish a number of booklets which are available directly from the Sports Council and they offer a hotline number (0171 383 2244) which athletes can telephone if they require a rapid response. In general, sports organisations tend to use the IOC list of prohibited substances but the regulations may vary from sport to sport and ultimately the onus is on the athlete to be aware of the regulations enforced by their own governing body. Providing a comprehensive list of banned substances for every sport is difficult. While guidelines are helpful the only certain method is for an athlete not to take any medication at all unless they have established officially beforehand that it is permitted. A doctor must also be careful not to prescribe a prohibited substance. If an athlete is detected using a prohibited substance, ignorance is no excuse for either athlete or doctor.

An athlete must be especially careful of drugs and medications bought 'over the counter'. The commonly available treatments for nasal congestion, catarrh and upper respiratory tract infections often contain banned substances. They are an effective treatment and do not have an ergogenic effect in therapeutic doses but they are prohibited because large doses have been abused by athletes. Other common pain relief preparations are similarly prohibited. Because these are bought over the counter, this is no guarantee that they are permitted in sport. Athletes, in their quest for that extra edge, are attracted by claims made on behalf some dietary supplements, vitamin preparations and tonic products reputed to restore energy. These may contain prohibited substances, especially if these products are purchased abroad, because regulations in respect of labelling and lists of contents may not be complete or accurate. Commonly available 'over the counter' preparations that are known to contain a prohibited substance include Bronchipax, Contac 400, Mucron, and Procol. Even the ubiquitous LemSip contains phenylephrine. These are just a few examples and there are many others.

Inclusion on a list of prohibited drugs does not automatically mean that this drug has a positive effect on performance. Detecting drug abuse is difficult, even using modern technological advances and some drugs are prohibited, not because of their own ergogenic effect them but because their metabolites are similar to those of a prohibited drugs and analysis cannot detect the difference.

The extent of the problem

The media discussion and extensive exposure given to the problems of drug abuse may lead us to believe that drug abuse is widespread. We do not, however, know the prevalence of drug abuse in sport. We have information about the number of positive tests detected by the Sports Council's London testing laboratory and, although the numbers are small, we should be alarmed by the rising numbers. Drug testing results from major sports events can also help us understand the magnitude of the problem. Remember, of course, that those detected have been foolish enough to get caught, that these are training drugs, and that they should have been stopped long before competition if the athlete wished to avoid detection. At the Olympics in Los Angeles [2] a banned drug was detected in just under 2% of 1,510 samples while at the Asian Games [3] 2 years later 3.2% of the samples contained a prohibited drug. Prohibited substances have also been detected at the Pan American games [4]. From 1986 to 1991 there were positive tests in 5.5% of 2,066 urine specimens collected from competitors in South Africa [5].

Summary of Reports from the Testing Programme

Class	1993/94	1994/95	1995/96	1996/97
Stimulants	11	30	41	40
Narcotics	5	4	4	1
Anabolic Agents	20	23	15	27
Diuretics	–	2	1	3
Peptide Hormones and Analogues	2	–	–	1
Alcohol	1	–	3	2
Marijuana	2	10	10	2
Beta-blockers	–	1	–	–
Hypnotic Sedatives	–	–	–	1
Refusal	6	7	15	13
Number of Reports	**47**	**77**	**89**	**90**
Number of Cases Reported	**43**	**67**	**84**	**82**

Key:
Reports – each report is for a finding of a prohibited substance or method, a refusal or non availability
Case – each case relates to one athlete and may contain more than one report
Reproduced with permission from the UK Sports Council, Ethics and Anti-Doping Directorate Annual Report, 1996/97

While we have little accurate prevalence data in the UK there are some very alarming figures for the prevalence of steroid use among adolescents the USA [6–8] where figures vary from 3% to 7.6%. Even Human Growth Hormone (HGH) abuse seems to be a problem in high schools [9] where 5% of males reported past or present use of HGH.

It appears that the problem of drug abuse in the UK is greatest among bodybuilders and a number of studies have shown interesting results. In a study of anabolic steroids in private gymnasia in Wales [10] 38.8% admitted to having taken steroids, while in Scotland [11], 19.5% of bodybuilders had used drugs. In the USA [12] 54% of men were using steroids on a regular basis compared to 10% of women competitors. Random, unannounced drugs tests probably give a more accurate measure of drug abuse and in such a study of body builders in Flanders [13] during 1988–1993 between 38 and 58% of those tested were found positive.

What do the athletes think?

It is very difficult to get an accurate view of the athlete's perspective on drug abuse. Surveys may not tell the whole story. The Sports Council surveyed 468 athletes [14] in 1995. Most of them had been tested (74%) and two-thirds (66%) expected to be tested in the following 12 months but many still felt that more testing was needed. They thought that testing was a deterrent but that it was not widespread enough to be a sufficient deterrent.

In a similar survey, 82% of Italian athletes [15] would like stricter controls not only during competitions but also during training. They believed (70%) that access to illegal substances was not difficult.

The drug testing procedure

Drug testing is undertaken on a urine sample. This has limitations. It is relatively imprecise, it cannot be used accurately to detect the presence of some drugs and is open to manipulation. There is some international pressure to change to a blood sample but this is unlikely to occur in the forseeable future. Because the testing procedure is open to manipulation and there is a need for a secure chain of transport between the testing station and the laboratory, the entire operation must conform to a very strict protocol.

The first stage of the procedure is notifying the athlete. Testing may occur at a competition or as an out of competition random test and those administering the test must now be accredited testing officials. These are known as Independent Sampling Officers and are trained and appointed by the UK Sports Council. They each carry a time-limited identity card and a letter of authority for the event to which they are allocated. The official notifies the athlete who must attend the testing station within a specified period of time. The athlete to be tested is asked to sign a form acknowledging this notification. The athlete then attends for testing but they may be accompanied by an official, and indeed must be accompanied if under 16 years of age. The testing area may be a dedicated mobile testing station or a temporary arrangement in a leisure centre or stadium. The testing area should have a waiting area which is private, comfortable and well supplied with sealed drinks.

The procedure for giving the sample, placing it in the appropriate bottles and sealing the bottles is highly regulated. The entire procedure is organised to ensure that the sample given by the athlete actually comes from that athlete and arrives at the laboratory without any opportunity for tampering with the sample. The athlete to be tested completes some duplicate forms, on which they have the opportunity to declare any drugs or medication taken in the previous 3 days. They are then offered the opportunity to choose their own numbered sample bottles and numbered seals. When giving the sample the athlete must be observed closely to ensure that the urine comes from the meatus. Approximately 100 ml is required. The athlete then signs to confirm that the procedure has been adhered to correctly, that the sample has been taken and placed in the bottles and tagged correctly, and they are given a copy of the paperwork. The sample is then sent for analysis. There are a limited number (currently 24) of laboratories accredited by the International Olympic Committee and there must be a secure line of transport to the laboratory.

If the sample tests positive the laboratory must notify the governing body of the particular sport, which then notifies the athlete. Each sport has its own procedure for dealing with positive tests but in all cases the athlete has a right to have a second analysis of the sample and to have a representative present at this analysis. With confirmation of this positive test, the athlete is offered the opportunity to present their case at a special hearing. While the procedure should be secure and straightforward a number of athletes have successfully appealed against positive tests in the past.

The testing procedure can be quite stressful for an athlete, especially those young and inexperienced and who may be attending their first major event abroad but many people are very uncomfortable giving a urine sample under observation. Unfortunately the procedure must be very rigorous to prevent abuse and efforts by athletes to confound the tests. There can be difficulties for athletes attempting to give a sample other than psychological stress. Those who have just completed an endurance event, perhaps in a hot environment, may be dehydrated and require considerable fluid replacement and time before a sample is available. Others may be deliberately dehydrated if attempting to make a weight in sports such as boxing, judo or rowing. If they have to compete on the following day they may be reluctant to drink knowing that they may have difficulty making the weight again.

Efforts can be made at various stages of the sampling procedure to alter the sample. It is possible to manipulate urinary excretion by taking medication to alter urinary PH or to block urinary excretion. Athletes can also physically manipulate the sample by catheterising themselves and instilling other urine. There are also other documented efforts to confound the system such as attempting to substitute the sample by urine from another source stored in a condom or catheter. Methods to confound the testing procedure are easier for women athletes. The regulations state that the testing officer must be able to see the urine issue from the meatus and pass into the bottle but there is a natural reluctance and embarrassment to watch the athlete too closely which plays into the hands of those trying to cheat the system. Those being tested must also ensure that the testing procedure is adhered to correctly. It is important that their sample is placed in the correct bottle and that the paperwork is completed correctly. The testing area can be very busy with athletes and officials but it is in the interests of the testing officer and all involved that the procedure is adhered to quickly and efficiently.

Out of competition testing is increasingly common. Most of the currently abused drugs are training drugs so that the athlete gains maximum benefit from their use outside the competition period. For this reason elite athletes are subject to year round random testing. In theory this is random unannounced testing, but there are, of course, logistical difficulties and the athlete may have prior warning of testing. If the athlete is training abroad the difficulties are confounded and it may be difficult to track down the top athletes who are often international globetrotters moving from one warm weather training venue to the next. In these circumstances it is impossible to undertake true random drug testing.

Classes of banned substances

The classes of drugs prohibited by the IOC are shown below and a regularly updated list is published in the BNF. All mechanical and chemical manipulation is prohibited together with many drugs considered to be ergogenic aids. These are divided into the following categories.

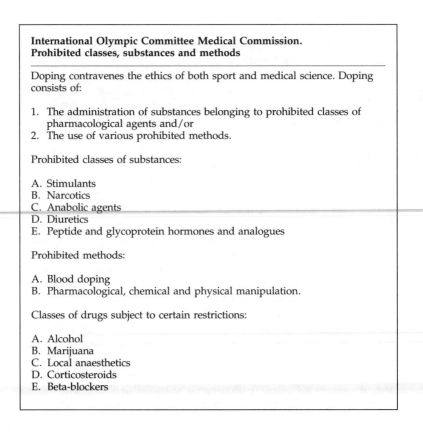

International Olympic Committee Medical Commission.
Prohibited classes, substances and methods

Doping contravenes the ethics of both sport and medical science. Doping consists of:

1. The administration of substances belonging to prohibited classes of pharmacological agents and/or
2. The use of various prohibited methods.

Prohibited classes of substances:

A. Stimulants
B. Narcotics
C. Anabolic agents
D. Diuretics
E. Peptide and glycoprotein hormones and analogues

Prohibited methods:

A. Blood doping
B. Pharmacological, chemical and physical manipulation.

Classes of drugs subject to certain restrictions:

A. Alcohol
B. Marijuana
C. Local anaesthetics
D. Corticosteroids
E. Beta-blockers

Drugs of abuse

Stimulants include all drugs related to amphetamines. They have a stimulant effect and are used to increase aggression and reduce fatigue. While they may be used in sports where explosive power is required, they are also used in endurance sports, especially cycling, to overcome fatigue at the end of a long stage. They have side-effects. They increase aggression, but may also increase anxiety and raise blood pressure. They may also cause arrythmias. One major concern is their addictive potential, but athletes are less concerned about this.

Sympathomimetic amines including ephedrine, pseudoephedrine, phenylpropranolamine and norpseudoephedrine are also prohibited but their importance is that they are found in nasal decongestants and cough suppressants and are a common cause of inadvertent positive tests. It is doubtful if they have a significant effect on performance. Caffeine [16] is also a stimulant and, much to the surprise of many, is a prohibited drug. Because of its widespread use it is subject to a threshold level so that it is only prohibited when the level of caffeine in the urine exceeds 12 µg l^{-1}.

Narcotic analgesics reduce pain sensitivity. In theory they could allow an athlete to continue in spite of injury but it is unlikely that their use would improve performance. The IOC doping regulations now permit codeine, dihydrocodeine and pholcodine but dextropropoxyphene remains a prohibited substance.

Anabolic steroids are probably the best known performance enhancing drugs. These are essentially training drugs and allow athletes to undertake greater training loads with improved recovery. The side-effects are known and well documented. They include both physical and psychological problems. Physical problems recorded in case reports include, rupture of the musculocutaneous junction, gynaecomastia, hypogonadism, alteration of the coagulation system, changes in lipid and lipoprotein subfractions, cholestasis, skin disease, hypertension, stroke and myocardial infarction. More modern preparations have improved anabolic effect with reduced androgenic effect so that some of the early signs of steroid abuse such as hypogonadism and baldness are less common.

Anabolic steroids improve strength and muscle mass and have been used by power athletes, weightlifters and bodybuilders. They have another and important effect which increases their potential for abuse by endurance athletes: improved recovery from training loads. The doses taken by power athletes and bodybuilders are huge and they often take several different types of anabolic steroid together, known as stacking, or use different steroids in cycles. The total dose may be 10–100 times the normal replacement equivalent of testosterone [17]. Taking these huge doses of anabolic steroids may make the athlete very aggressive, known in the sporting community as 'roid rage' but they may also be subject to severe depression between drug cycles.

These drugs are used mainly as training aids, so that athletes preparing for a major competition can plan their drug cycle to be drug free well before competition. If they time it correctly their drug use should be undetectable at the time of the event. There are over 100 anabolic steroids available, some taken orally and some given by injection, and athletes use cocktails of these drugs to maximum effect. If they know how long it takes before their use of each product is undetectable they can plan their use as close as possible to the event. They may take other medications at the same time such as diuretics to reduce fluid retention, thyroxine to promote weight loss, and tamoxifen to prevent gynaecomastia.

Testosterone is a naturally occurring anabolic steroid and it is difficult to determine abuse simply because of a greater than expected level of a naturally occurring hormone. Testosterone is, however, produced naturally in the body together with epitestosterone. The crude level of testosterone is not therefore used alone but the drug test depends on the testosterone–epitestosterone ratio. A ratio of greater than 6:1 is deemed positive.

There has been recent publicity about the use of β-2 agonists in the beef industry, where it is used for its anabolic effect to improve lean body weight. Clenbuterol (or angel dust as it is known in the beef industry) is prohibited. Other β-2 agonists are also prohibited although salbutamol, salmeterol and terbutaline, are permitted by inhalation, although they must be declared. They are not allowed for systemic use.

Testing for anabolic steroids is still not definitive and there are doubts about the possibility of false positive tests [18]. One interesting piece of research suggested that it may be possible to produce a positive drug test from ingesting meat from steroid-treated livestock [19]. Anabolic steroids are quite freely available in many local fitness clubs and leisure centres. General practitioners may be asked about the hazards and side-effects of these drugs and may even be asked by patients to monitor them for adverse side-effects.

Beta-blockers can be used as aids to performance. Clearly they will impair endurance performance, but it is this very effect in reducing heart rate and the systemic effects of anxiety that make them most effective in events where control of anxiety and heart rate is important. The benefits are greatest in events such as shooting [20] and archery, to produce bradycardia where the athlete who tries to shoot between heart beats has greater opportunity. Clearly they are also of potential benefit in sports such as bowls, darts and golf. Other sports in which the use of β-blockers is banned include: bobsleigh and luge, ski-jumping and free style skiing, diving and synchronised swimming and modern pentathlon.

Diuretics are banned, not because of any potential ergogenic effect but because they may be abused by athletes attempting to lose weight to compete in a weight category or to increase volume and dilution of a urine sample to confound the drug test.

Peptide hormones are now known as the sports designer drugs, because they can be used without detection. Growth hormone (HGH, somatotrophin) has an anabolic effect and athletes can use it without fear of detection. Early growth hormone preparations were of human origin and there is still some fear among ex-athletes that they may have been infected with Creutzfeldt–Jacob disease. Human chorionic gonadotrophin (HCG) is used to increase the production of endogenous steroids, particularly testosterone. Its attraction to athletes is that it stimulates both testosterone and epitestosterone production. Corticotrophin (ACTH) increases the level of endogenous corticosteroids and may alter mood. It is a prohibited drug, although its ergogenic potential is minimal.

Endurance athletes will benefit from improvements in oxygen carrying capacity, hence the experiments with blood doping. Blood doping, which is prohibited, is effective [21], but exceptionally difficult to detect. Because it involves taking a large volume of blood, and storing it for later reinfusion, it carries a risk. Erythropoietin has been used by endurance athletes to gain exactly the same benefit by increasing haematocrit. The use of erythropoietin is banned but undetectable.

The regulations also state that pharmacological, chemical and physical manipulation of the drug testing procedure is prohibited. This includes physical methods described above to tamper with the urine testing procedure but also includes drugs used to alter renal excretion. This includes drugs such as Probenecid and related substances which have no ergogenic effect themselves.

Administration of epitestosterone to correct the ratio to testosterone in the urine is also prohibited.

Alcohol, marijuana and local anaesthetics are subject to special conditions. Some local anaesthetics are allowed for local or intra-articular use, but there must be prior notification to the relevant medical authority and then only when medically justified. Corticosteroids are permitted for topical use, by inhalation and by intra-articular and local injection and then only with written notification to the relevant medical authority.

It is very unlikely that any long-term solution will be found to the problem of drug abuse in sport. Athletes have always sought that extra advantage and it seems that the testing technology stays one step behind those using performance enhancing drugs. There is no solution. We cannot detect the modern peptide hormones and those who have enough money can clearly abuse these medications with impunity. Even for those taking drugs that can be detected, the chances of detection are minimal if they approach it in a calculated manner. If they are caught, the penalties are unlikely to act as a major deterrent.

References

1 MacAuley D. Drug abuse in sport. *BMJ*. 1996; **313**: 211–14.
2 Catlin DH, Kammerer RC, Hatton CK *et al*. Analytical chemistry at the Games of the XXIIIrd Olympiad in Los Angeles 1984. *Clin Chem* 1987; **33**: 319–27.
3 Park J. Doping test report of 10th Asian Games in Seoul. *J Sports Med Phys Fitness*. 1991; **31**: 303–17.
4 Wagner JC, Ulrich LR, McKean DC, Blankenbaker RG. Pharmaceutical services at the Tenth Pan American Games. *Am J Hosp Pharm* 1989; **46**: 2023–7.
5 van der Merwe PJ, Kruger HS. Drugs in sport – results of the past 6 years of dope testing. *S Afr Med J* 1992; **82**: 151–3.
6 Whitehead R, Chillag S, Elliott D. Anabolic steroid use among adolescents in a rural state. *J Fam Prac* 1992; **35**: 401–5.
7 Terney R, McLain LG. The use of anabolic steroids in high school students. *Am J Dis Child* 1990; **144**: 99–103.
8 Windsor R, Dumitru D. Prevalence of anabolic steroid use by male and female adolescents. *Med Sci Sports Exer* 1989; **21**: 494–7.
9 Rickert VI, Pawlak-Morello C., Sheppard V, Jay MS. Human growth hormone: a new substance of abuse among adolescents? *Clin Pediatr* 1992; **31**: 723–6.
10 Perry HM, Wright D, Littlepage BN. Dying to be big: a review of anabolic steroid use. *Br J Sports Med* 1992; **26**: 259–61.
11 McKillop G. Drug abuse in body builders in the West of Scotland. *Scot Med J* 1987; **32**: 39–41.
12 Tricker R, O'Neill MR, Cook D. The incidence of anabolic steroid use among competitive bodybuilders. *J Drug Edu* 1989; **19**: 313–25.

13 Delbeke FT, Desmet N, Debackere M. The abuse of doping agents in competing body builders in Flanders. (1988–1993). *Int J Sports Med* 1995; **16**: 66–70.

14 *Doping Control in the UK.* A survey of the experiences and views of elite competitors 1995. Sports Council, London, 1995.

15 Scarpino V, Arrigo A, Benzi G, *et al.* Evaluation of prevalence of 'doping' among Italian athletes. *Lancet* 1990; **336**: 1048–50.

16 Spriet LL. Caffeine and performance. *Int J Sport Nutr*. 1995; 5 (Suppl): S84–99.

17 Goldberg L. Adverse effects of anabolic steroids. *JAMA* 1996 **276**: 257.

18 Raynaud E, Audran M, Brun JF *et al.* False-positive cases in detection of testosterone doping. *Lancet* 1992; **340**: 1468–9.

19 Kicman AT, Cowan DA, Myhre L *et al.* Effect on sports drug tests of ingesting meat from steroid (methenolone)-treated livestock. *Clin Chem* 1994; **40**: 2084–7.

20 Kruse P, Ladefoged J, Paulev PE *et al.* Beta-blockade used in precision sports: effects on pistol shooting performance. *J Appl Physiol* 1986; **61**: 417–20.

21 Berglund B, Hemmingson P. Effect of reinfusion of autologus blood on exercise performance in cross-country skiers. *Int J Sports Med* 1987; **8**: 231–3.

Appendix: useful addresses

British Journal of Sports Medicine
BMA House
Tavistock Square
London WC1 9JR

British Association of Sport and Medicine
Secretary John Clegg
Birch Lea
67 Springfield Lane
Eccleston, St Helens
Merseyside WA10 5HB

British Olympic Association
Medical Director
Dr Richard Budgett
1 Wandsworth Plain
London SW18 1HE

British Olympic Medical Centre
Nothwick Park Hospital
Watford Road
Harrow, Middlesex HA1 3UJ

Institute of Sports Medicine
at University College London Medical School
Charles Bell House
67–73 Riding House Street
London W1P 7LD

Scottish Institute of Sports Medicine and Sports Science
University of Strathclyde
Jordanhill Campus
76 Southbrae Drive
Glasgow G13 1PP

United Kingdom Sports Council
16 Upper Woburn Place
London WC1H 0QP

Educational courses

Bath Distance Learning Course
Malcolm Bottomley
Course Medical Director
University of Bath Sports Medicine Course for Doctors
University of Bath
Bath BA2 7AY

Lister Postgraduate Institute
The Postgraduate Dean
The Lister postgraduate Institute
11 Hill Square
Edinburgh EH8 9DR

National Sports Medicine Institute/BASM
Medical College of St Bartholomews Hospital
Charterhouse Square
London EC1M 6BQ

Royal Society of Medicine
Section of Sports Medicine
1 Wimpole Street
London W1M 8AE

Society of Orthopaedic Medicine
Course Organiser
Society of Orthopaedic Medicine
1 The Mall
Faversham
Kent ME13 8JL

Postgraduate qualifications to Masters level

Glasgow University
Dept of Sports Medicine
Institute of Biomedical and Life Sciences
64 Oakfield Ave
Glasgow G12 8LB

Royal London Hospital Medical College
Department of Sports Medicine
Mann Ward
Royal London Hospital (Mile End)
Bancroft Road
London E2 4DG

University of Nottingham Medical School
Course Administrator
Centre for Sports Medicine
Orthopaedic and Accident Surgery
C Floor, West Block
Queens Medical Centre
Nottingham NG7 2UH

Trinity College, Dublin
Department of Anatomy
Trinity College
Dublin 2

Diploma examinations in sports medicine

Society of Apothecaries Diploma in Sports Medicine
The Registrar
Society of Apothecaries
Blackfriars Lane
London EC4V 6EJ

Scottish Royal College Diploma Examination in Sports Medicine
Royal Colleges Board Secretary
Royal College of Surgeons at Edinburgh
Nicholson Street
Edinburgh EH8 9DW

International addresses

ACSM
American College of Sports Medicine
Box 1440
Indianapolis
IN 46206–1440
USA

AMSSM
American Medical Society for Sports Medicine
7611 Elmwood Ave, Suite 202
Middleton, WI 53562
USA

Australian College of Sports Physicians
PO Box 644
Crows Nest
New South Wales 2065
Australia

CASM
Canadian Academy of Sports Medicine
Suite 502
R Tait Mc Kenzie Building
1600 James Naismith Drive
Gloucester ON K1B 5N4
Canada

European Federation of Sports Medicine
Professor G. Giodano-Lanza
President
urf de Médicine
74 Rue Léonardo de Vinci
F–93012
Bobigny Cedex
France

FIMS
Fédération Internationale de Médecine du Sport
Spaulding Rehabilitation Hospital
125 Nashau Street
Boston MA 02114-1198
USA

Index

Abdominal injuries, 124
Abrasions, 232
Acclimatisation
    to altitude, 199, 208
    to heat, 199–202
Acetazolamide, 208
Acromio-clavicular joint
    dislocation, 115
    injection, 178
Adductor muscles (leg)
    groin strain, 128
    stretches, 79, 81
Aerobic exercise, 49
Aerobic metabolism, 46–7
Altitude sickness, 199, 206–8
Amenorrhoea, 238–9
Amnesia, 101
Amphetamines, 265
Anaerobic metabolism, 45–6, 47
Anaesthetics, local, 268
Analgesics
    for minor injuries, 72
    narcotic, 265
Ankle
    examination, 157–9
    sprain, 160–2
        chronic, 164–5
    taping, 173
Anorexia, 223
Antioxidants, 254
Apprehension test, 113
Arthritis, 55
Asthma, 212–14
Athlete's foot, 230

Back pain, 104
    acute injuries, 106–7
    children, 109–10
    chronic injuries, 107–9
    examination, 104–6

Back stretches, 79, 82
Baker's cyst, 153
Beta-2 agonists, 266
Beta-blockers, 55, 267
Blisters, 233
Blood doping, 267
Blood pressure and exercise, 19
Bodybuilders and drug abuse, 261
Bone density in women, 238, 239–40
Boxing and head injuries, 99
Brain ischaemia, 100
Breast cancer, 225, 240
Bronchospasm, exercise induced,
    213–14
Burns, friction, 234
Bursitis, 152
    iliopsoas, 130
    pes anserinus, 178
    prepatellar, 178
    subacromial, 116
    trochanteric, 126, 130, 178

Caffeine, 265
Calf stretches, 77, 78
Cancer, 225
    breast, 225, 240
    and exercise, 11
Carbohydrates, 247–8, 249
    loading, 48, 249–50
    meals around events, 252–3
Cardiac adaptation to exercise, 43, 94–5
Cardiac hypertrophy, 91
Cardiomyopathy, hypertrophic
    pre-exercise screening, 91–2
    and sudden death, 89, 90
Cardiovascular disease and exercise,
    11–12, 12–15
    blood pressure, 19
    cardiac rehabilitation, 36–7, 94
    effect of drugs, 35–6

energy expenditure, 15–16
fibrinogen, 19–20
lifestyle modification, 36
lipids, 18
physical fitness, 17
protective level of activity, 20–1
sudden death *see* Death, sudden
   cardiac
Carpal tunnel syndrome, 177
Cerebral oedema at altitude, 207
Children and exercise, 64–6
back problems, 109–10
risks, 66–9
China, exercise and medicine in
   ancient, 2
Cholesterol, 18
Chromosome testing, 244–5
Chronic fatigue syndrome, 221
'Cinema' sign, 151
Clarke's sign, 151
Clavicle fracture, 114–15
Clenbuterol, 266
Compartment syndromes, 156–7
Compression after soft tissue injuries,
   72
Concussion, 98, 101
Contusions, 74
Corticosteroid use, 268
injections, 119, 172–9
Corticotrophin, 267
Cough, exercise related, 214
Creatine, 255
Cruciate ligaments
anterior
   assessment, 140, 141–2
   injuries, 143, 144–7
posterior, 140
Cycling
back pain, 108–9
hamstring tendinitis, 136
helmets, 99
impotence, 125
metabolism issues, 47
numbness of hand, 122
Cyst, Baker's, 153

Dark Ages and physical education, 5
de Quervain disease, 121
'Dead leg', 74
Death, sudden cardiac, 86–7, 88–9
prevention, 87–8
risk estimation, 89–91, 92–4

Dehydration, 201–2
prevention, 202–3
weight category sports, 201, 255
Depression, 224
Diabetes mellitus, 216–18
Diarrhoea
in runners, 225–6
traveller's, 196–7, 226
Diet, 247–51
carbohydrate loading, 48, 249–50
fluid balance, 255
meals around events, 252–3
supplements, 253–5
weight reduction, 251–2
Dislocations
acromio-clavicular, 115
finger, 122
shoulder, 113
Diuretics, 55, 267
Doctors, team
legal responsibilities, 189–91
medical bag, 187–9
responsibilities, 180–1
Doping, blood, 267
Douching, vaginal, 125
Drawer sign, ankle, 159
Drawer test, knee, 140, 141
Drugs, performance enhancing, 257–8
banned substances, 258–9, 264–8
drug testing, 261–4
extent of problem, 260–1

Eczema, 232
Effusion, knee, 138
Elbow injuries, 118–20
Elevation after minor injuries, 72
Emergencies, 85
see also Death, sudden cardiac
Endurance sports
diabetes control, 217
glycogen stores, 250
Endurance training, 52, 56
Energy threshold for cardiovascular
   benefits, 15–16
Ephedrine, 265
Epicondylitis
lateral *see* Tennis elbow
medial *see* Golfer's elbow
Epilepsy, 218
Erythropoietin, 267
Events management, major sporting,
   181–4

Exercise
  for children *see* Children and exercise
  current population activity levels,
    21–2, 64–5
  effect on lipids, 18
  historical perspective, 1–9
  medical benefits, 5–7, 11–12
  see also Cardiovascular disease and
    exercise
  for older people *see* Older people and
    exercise
Exercise prescription schemes, 29–31,
  33–4

Fartlek training, 52
Fat, dietary, 24–89
Fat, proportions of body, 237–8
Fatty acid metabolism, 47
Femur
  fractures, 129–30
  trochanteric bursitis, 126, 130
Fibrinogen and exercise, 19–20
Finger injuries, 122–3
  taping, 173
Finkelstein's test, 121
Fitness
  and cardiovascular disease, 17
  current levels in older people, 56–7
  measuring, 49–52
Flexor tendinitis, 168
Fluid balance, 201, 255
  dehydration, 201–2
  fluid replacement, 202–3
Foot
  abnormalities, 169–70
  injuries, 166–9
Footwear, 170–1
Form, loss of, 221
Fractures
  clavicle, 114–15
  femur, 129–30
  foot, 166, 169
  march, 166
  metatarsal, 166, 169
  pars interarticularis, 107–8
  pubic ramus, 129
  stress, 129–30, 153–5, 166
    treatment, 155–6
  wrist, 120
Framingham heart study, 14
Friction burns, 234
Frostbite, 209–10

Fungal skin infections, 230

Galen on exercise, 3–4
Gamekeeper's thumb, 122
Gender testing, 243–5
Genital injuries, 124–6
'Gilmore's groin', 127
Ginseng, 254
Glandular fever, 220–1
Glasgow coma scale, 100
Glycogen, 46–7, 48, 249–50
Golfer's elbow, 120, 177
Gravel rash, 234
Greece, exercise in ancient, 2–4
Groin pain, 127–30
Growth hormone, 267
Growth plate injuries, 67
Gymnastics and back pain, 109

Haematoma
  intracranial, 100
  subungual, 233
Haematuria, 125–6
Haemoglobin, 251
Haemoglobinuria, 125–6
Haemorrhages, retinal, 207
Hamstring injuries, 132–6
Hamstring stretches, 77–9
Hand grip strength, 57
Hand injuries, 121–3
Harvard alumni study, 14
Head injuries, 98–100
  advice to patients, 101–2
  concussion, 98, 101
Head protection, 99
Headaches, 218–19
Heart *see* Cardiac
Heat and humidity acclimatisation,
  199–201, 203–5
Heel injuries, 167, 179
Hepatitis A, 222
Hepatitis B, 222
Hernias, 127–8
Herpes simplex, 231
Hip
  examination, 126–7
  pain, 127–30
History of exercise, 1–5
  early studies on benefits, 5–7
'Hitting the wall', 47, 249
HIV infection, 222

Hormones, peptide, 267
Human chorionic gonadotrophin, 267
Hyperpronation of feet, 168–9
Hypertension, 19
Hyperthermia, 202
Hypothermia, 208–9

Ice treatment, 71, 118–19
Iliotibial band
  corticosteroid injection, 178
  friction syndrome, 151
Immune system and exercise, 220,
  224–5
Immunisations, 193–4
Impact heel, 167
Impetigo, 231
Impotence in cyclists, 125
Independent Sampling Officers, 262
Infectious diseases
  prevention, 223
  skin infections, 230–1
  training grounds and, 221–2
  traveller's diarrhoea, 196–7, 226
  viral illnesses, 219–21, 222
Infectious mononucleosis, 220–1
Information leaflets
  anterior knee pain, 148–50
  exercise for older people, 60–2
Injections, corticosteroid *see under*
  Corticosteroid use
Injuries from sport
  in children, 67–8
  history checklist, 83–4
  soft tissue, 70–4
  spinal *see* Back pain; Spine injuries
  see also Emergencies; *specific body
    parts*
Iron, dietary, 251

Jet lag, 194–6
Jock itch, 230
'Jogger's nipple', 232

Knee
  anterior pain, 147–51
  effusion, 138
  examination, 137–43
  extensor strength, 57
  'giving way', 144
  ligaments, 139–42

'locking', 143–4

Lacerations, 234–5
Lachman's test, 140, 142
Lactic acid, 51–2
Leg extensor power, 57
Legal responsibilities of team doctors,
  189–91
Ligaments
  ankle, 158
  collateral (knee), 139
  cruciate *see* Cruciate ligaments
Lipids and exercise, 18

Mackenzie, James, 7
Mallet finger, 122–3
Marathon runners' metabolism, 47
Marathons: medical planning, 182–3
Marfans syndrome, 90
Mass participation events: medical
  issues, 182–3
McCleod guidelines on doctors'
  responsibilites, 190–1
Medial plica syndrome, 151
Medial tibial stress syndrome, 157
Medical bag and equipment, 187–9
Medical examination
  pre-exercise, 37–40, 184–6
  cardiac screening, 87, 88, 91–2,
    95–6
  pre-tour, 186–7
  transfer, 187
Medications
  older people, 54–5
  'over the counter', 227, 259
  see also Drugs, performance
    enhancing
Melatonin, 195
Meniscus injury, 143
Menstrual cycle and exercise, 238,
  242
Metabolism during exercise, 45–7
Metatarsalgia, 170
Migraine, 218–19
Minerals, 251
Misoprostol, 73
Motivation to exercise, 31–3
Mountain pursuits
  altitude sickness, 206–8
  frostbite, 209–10
  hypothermia, 208–9

Muscle
  age-related changes, 54
  changes after training, 43
  contusions, 74
  fibre types, 45
  soreness, 73
  tears, thigh, 131, 133–5
Myocardial infarction and exercise, 93
Myocarditis, viral, 88
Myositis ossificans, 74

Narcotic analgesics, 265
Neck stretches, 82
Neuroma, interdigital, 169–70
Neuropraxia, ulnar nerve, 122
Nipple abrasions, 232
Noble compression test, 151
Non-steroidal anti-inflammatory
    medications, 72

Obesity, 65, 227–8
Occupation and cardiovascular disease,
    7–8, 13–14
Oedema, pulmonary and cerebral, at
    altitude, 207
Older people and exercise, 53
  age-related changes, 54
  assessing risks, 58–9
  illness and medication, 54–5
  information leaflet, 60–2
  osteoporosis, 239–40
  preventing sudden cardiac death,
    87–8
  types of exercise, 55–6
Osgood-Schlatter disease, 152–3
Osteitis pubis, 129
Osteoarthritis, 215–16
Osteochondritis dessicans, 153
Osteoporosis, 238, 239–40
Oxygen saturation at altitude, 206
Oxygen uptake measurement, 49–51

PACE programme, 34–5
Pars interarticularis fracture, 107–8
Patella taping, 173
Performance limits, 8–9
Physical activity definition, 16–17
Physician-based Assessment and
    Counselling for Exercise, 34–5
Physiology of exercise
  cardiac adaptation, 43, 94–5

  metabolism, 45–7
  muscle adaptation, 43
  performance prediction tests, 45,
    49–52
Physiotherapy, 75
Pivot shift test, 140
Plantar fasciitis, 167, 179
'Policeman's heel', 167, 179
Pregnancy, 242–3
Proprioceptive Neuromuscular
    Rehabilitation, 76
Protein in diet, 248
Pseudoephedrine, 265
Psoriasis, 232
Psychological factors
  motivation to exercise, 31–3, 34
  and training, 44–5
Puberty and exercise, 66–7
Pulmonary oedema at altitude, 207

'Q' angle, 138, 237
Quadriceps
  injuries, 131–2
  and knee pain, 148–9
  stretches, 79, 80

Radius, fracture of, 120
Rectus femoris tear, 131–2
Rehabilitation
  anterior cruciate ligament injury, 145–6
  cardiac, 94
  hamstring tears, 134–5
  see also Stretching
Resistance training in older people, 56,
    58
Respiratory disease, 211–14
Rest
  following corticosteroid injections,
    176
  following minor injuries, 71
Resuscitation, role of cardiopulmonary,
    86
Retinal haemorrhages at altitude, 207
Rhinitis, allergic, 227
RICE, 71–2
'Roid rage', 266
Roman Empire and exercise, 4–5
Rotator cuff injuries, 115–16
Rowing
  back pain, 108
  fluid balance in lightweights, 255

studies on medical benefits, 5–7
Running, and haematuria, 125

Scaphoid fracture, 120
Scheuermann's disease, 110
Second injury syndrome, 73
Sex chromatin test, 244
Shin splints, 153
Shoes, sports, 170–1
Shoulder
  examination, 111–13, 114
  injection of joint, 116, 117, 178
  injuries, 111–16
    management, 116–18
  stretches, 79, 82
Simmond's test, 164
Skier's thumb, 121–2
Skill, sporting, 44
Skin problems, 230–5
Smoking, 212
Sodium and fluid replacement, 203
Somatotrophin, 267
Speed, 44
Spine injuries
  cervical, 103–4
  see also Back pain
Spondylolysis, 107–8
Stamina, 44
Steroids
  anabolic, 265–6
  corticosteroids, 268
Stimulants:banned substances, 265
Strapping, 162, 172, 173, 174
Strength, 44
Stretching, 75–82
Subacromial bursitis, 116
Sun protection, 198, 233
Supplements, dietary, 253–5
Supraspinatus tendinitis, 116
Suturing lacerations, 234–5
Sweat rash, 233–4
Swelling after soft tissue injuries, 72
Sympathomimetic amines, 265
Symphisitis pubis, 128–9

Taping, 162, 172, 173, 174
Technological advances and athletic
  performance, 9
Temperature, wet bulb globe, 205
Tendinitis
  Achilles', 163

in foot, 168
hamstring, 136
supraspinatus, 116
Tendon, Achilles', 162–3
  examination, 157, 158, 159
  injuries, 163–4
Tennis elbow, 118–20, 177
Tenosynovitis, 121, 177
Tenovaginitis, 121
Testosterone, 266
Thigh injuries, 131–6
Thomas' test, 126–7
Thompson's test, 164
Thumb taping, 173
Tibial tap, 138
Ticks, 222–3
Tinea cruris, 230
Toenails, ingrowing, 235–6
Touring
  consultations, 196
  immunisations, 193–4
  planning, 193–4
  pre-tour medical examination, 186–7
  travel issues, 194–6
  traveller's diarrhoea, 196–7
  see also Acclimatisation
Toxocara canis, 222
Toxoplasmosis gondii, 221
Training, 42–3
  components, 43–5
  Fartlek, 52
  heat acclimatisation, 199–201,
    203–5
  in older people, 56, 58
  physiological effects, 43
  sport-specific, 48
Training camp consultations, 196
Training of Young Athletes (TOYA)
  study, 67–8
Transfer medical examinations, 187
Trendelenberg's test, 126
Trochanteric bursitis, 126
Turf toe, 169

Ulna fractures, 120
Ulnar nerve damage, 122
Urethral injuries, 125
Urine
  drug testing, 261–4
  monitoring fluid loss, 202
Urticaria, exercise-induced, 226–7

Vastus medialis obliquus and knee
    pain, 148–9
Verrucas, 231
Victorians and exercise, 5
Viral infections, 219–21
    and cardiac disease, 88
Vitamins, 250–1
    vitamin C, 254
VO₂max, 50–1
    age-related changes, 54
    in women, 241

Walking, 28–9
'Wall, hitting the', 47, 249
Warm-up, 75, 77
    for asthmatics, 214
    see also Stretching

Water skiing and vaginal douching,
    125
Weight (body)
    obesity, 65, 227–8
    reduction, 223, 251–2
    gauging fluid loss, 201
Whitehall study, 13–14
Wolff–Parkinson–White syndrome,
    90–1
Women
    athletic performance, 241
    menstrual cycle, 238, 242
        amenorrhoea, 238–9
    osteoporosis, 238, 239–40
    physical differences to men, 237–8
    pregnancy, 242–3
    see also Breast cancer
Wrist injuries, 120–1